Handbook for

Dental Identification

Techniques in Forensic Dentistry

Handbook for

Dental Identification

Techniques in Forensic Dentistry

by

Lester L. Luntz, D.D.S.

Lieutenant, State Police Surgeon
Bureau of Identification
Connecticut State Police
Consultant in Forensic Odontology to the Office of the Medical Examiner, State of Connecticut
Consultant to the Armed Forces Institute of Pathology
Walter Reed Army Medical Center
Washington, D.C.

and

Phyllys Luntz

17 92

J. B. Lippincott Company
Philadelphia and Toronto

ISBN 0-397-50315-6

Library of Congress Catalog Card Number 73-4304

Printed in the United States of America

4 3 2 1

Library of Congress Cataloging in Publication Data

Luntz, Lester L
Handbook for dental identification.

1. Dental jurisprudence. I. Luntz, Phyllys, joint author. II. Title. [DNLM: 1. Forensic dentistry. W 705 L964h 1973]
RA1062.L86 363.2′44 73-4304
ISBN 0-397-50315-6

Mona and Frank

"This above all, to thine own self be true,
And it must follow, as the night the day,
Thou canst not then be false to any man."

Foreword

Forensic dentistry is a rapidly growing field of professional activity which should be of vital interest and concern to everyone involved in official medical-legal investigation, including forensic pathologists, criminalists, law enforcement officials, and criminal trial lawyers, both prosecution and defense. The significant and dramatic changes that have occurred in the criminal justice system in the United States during the past decade have led to a greater recognition and need for the utilization of physical evidence and scientific data in homicides and other criminal cases. These rather revolutionary changes have generated a whole new surge of activity in the various forensic sciences, and have stimulated the rapid growth and development of many new interfaces between law and science.

Unfortunately, there have not been a sufficient number of educational programs in forensic dentistry in the United States, either in dental schools or at the postgraduate level. Likewise, the scientific literature is not replete with publications designed to teach the practicing dentist how to apply his professional training, background, and daily practice to legal processes in appropriate cases. Forensic scientists and police officers similarly have not had available a good, single publication which could answer the many questions and problems that confront them in murder cases, identification problems, and other criminal investigations in which expertise in the field of forensic dentistry is required.

The HANDBOOK FOR DENTAL IDENTIFICATION represents an excellent and badly needed contribution to the medical-legal and criminal investigation literature. It is concise, compact, detailed, and informative. The numerous photographs and other visual aids employed by the author enable the reader to easily and quickly grasp the many points that are made in the text. The articulate and smooth flowing style of this book will permit police officers who may have had no opportunity for formal training in the scientific fields to readily comprehend the enumerable, timely, and relevant items that the author has packed into this highly useful handbook.

Dr. Lester L. Luntz is one of the foremost forensic odontologists in the United States today. His educational background, practical experience, contributions to the scientific literature, and accomplishments in various professional organizations easily qualify him as an outstanding expert in this field. The author has been a practicing dentist for a quarter of a century, during which time he has constantly increased his interest and professional involvement in the challenging "super" specialty field of forensic dentistry. Perhaps more than any other forensic odontologist in the world, Dr. Luntz has developed a close working relationship as a professional consultant with numerous police agencies and various other law enforcement groups throughout his home state of Connecticut. He has lectured widely on many different aspects of this important subject, and he has always been extremely unselfish in expending time and effort to assist his fellow forensic scientists, police officers, attorneys, and governmental agencies in those criminal cases and other legal matters in which dental expertise was required.

The HANDBOOK FOR DENTAL IDENTIFICATION is a veritable wealth of valuable information which, fortunately, is presented in such a way as to be of immediate, practical benefit to police and medical-legal investigators. The many case histories that Dr. Luntz has taken from his own personal consultation files demonstrate in a dramatic and vivid fashion the importance and value of applying dental knowledge and skills to problems of identification of unknown bodies, homicide investigations, and other similar problems. Bitemark studies, special surgical techniques for adequate dental examination at autopsy, postmortem charting, special photographic and x-ray techniques, and the use of antemortem dental records and charts for comparison purposes are only some of the fascinating and valuable discussions to be found in this excellent text.

The HANDBOOK FOR DENTAL IDENTIFICATION will undoubtedly become a permanent fixture on the bookshelves of the offices of all Medical Examiners and Coroners, crime laboratories, Federal, State and local law enforcement investigative agencies, and forensic science libraries. It is a welcome addition to the medical-legal, law enforcement, and scientific literature. Because of the outstanding reputation, expertise, and acknowledged authoritativeness of the author, the textbook will be referred to and utilized by many attorneys and scientists in homicides and other criminal trials on many occasions in future years.

CYRIL H. WECHT, M.D., J.D., F.C.A.P.

Coroner, Allegheny County, Pennsylvania; Research Professor of Law and Director; Institute of Forensic Sciences, Duquesne University· Clinical Assistant Professor of Pathology, University of Pittsburgh School of Medicine; Director, Pittsburgh Institute of Legal Medicine; Past President, American Academy of Forensic Sciences; Past President, American College of Legal Medicine; Diplomate, American Board of Pathology (Anatomic, Clinical, and Forensic Pathology)

Foreword

The ever expanding population masses throughout the world bring us tremendous and growing identification chores. The magnitude of these tasks is greatly increased with the domestic and international mobility of today's people. Disasters that result in death—whether it be one death or hundreds—bring with them difficult and complicated identification problems. It is imperative, therefore, for law enforcement agencies to be as well prepared as possible to identify these dead.

The task of identifying victims of mass accidents is often turned over to the disaster squad of the FBI's Identification Division, whose cooperative efforts result in many positive identifications. Most often these identifications come through the recording of postmortem fingerprints and then comparing them with antemortem records on file in Washington. All too frequently, however, disaster victims are so burned or mutilated that identifiable fingerprints are not possible to obtain, and other means of identification must be tried. Probably the most productive of the other methods is dental identification, or forensic dentistry as it is sometimes called.

HANDBOOK FOR DENTAL IDENTIFICATION, while written primarily as a concise guide for practicing dentists who happen to become involved in this very specialized segment of personal identification, has a very definite place in law enforcement literature and should be included in the library of every identification bureau and crime detection laboratory. It is written in a manner that is clear to the average identification officer and it does not require a dental degree to understand the text. The Glossary of Dental Terms included in the appendix will clarify any technical words that are unfamiliar to the law enforcement officer.

The description of the dental identification kit in Chapter 3 will be of special interest to any department considering the formation of a dental identification unit. It is probably the first kit ever designed for dental identification work. Chapter 9, which covers the subject of bite-marks, should be of interest to all criminal investigators, any one of whom could become involved with such evidence without advance notice.

One of the authors, Dr. Lester L. Luntz, is a practicing dentist in Hartford, Connecticut, and also a lieutenant in the Connecticut State Police. To our knowledge, Dr. Luntz is the first dentist ever assigned to a law enforcement agency's identification bureau. In 1969 he formed the first Dental Sisaster Squad, composed of over 60 volunteer dentists, and in conjunction with that, in 1969 and 1970 he conducted the first symposiums on forensic dentistry in the United States. In 1973, in a landmark bite-mark case in Illinois, he became the first dentist to be issued a search warrant, authorizing him to take impressions and photographs of the mouth of a suspect.

Not a large book, the volume is compact and satisfies the requirements of a handbook. It is easily carried by a dentist or a police officer to the scene of a dental investigation.

T. Dickerson Cooke

Director, Institute of Applied Science, Chicago, Illinois. Editor, *Fingerprint and Identification Magazine,* Chicago, Illinois. Historian, International Association for Identification.

Preface

Dental identification has come of age. It has been evolving over the past twenty years, although its roots go far back in history. Identification of a human body is usually a prerequisite for estate settlement, payment of life insurance, remarriage by the surviving partner and prosecution in cases of homicide. Law enforcement agencies are coming to recognize the assistance that dentistry can render as a sophisticated tool for identification.

In this modern era of mobility, violence and traumatic death there is an increasing reliance upon the use of dental identification when other methods of identifying a victim cannot be employed. In disasters such as plane crashes, fires, floods, automobile accidents—whenever the body may have suffered decomposition, mutilation or incineration—visual identification, the most common means, or identification by fingerprints may not be possible. Moreover, even though fingerprints are obtainable, there may be no record of fingerprints on file.

It is a valid assumption that during their lifetime more people have been to a dentist than have had their fingerprints recorded. Significantly, the teeth are the least destructible part of the human body after death, while in life they are probably that part of the body most frequently attacked by disease. Caries (tooth-rot) is treated by the removal of the decay in the tooth structure and the insertion of restorations. Since restorations are also highly resistant to destruction after death, one can expect to recover from a body both the teeth and restorations.

The number of different combinations possible in charting the human mouth is astronomical. On that is founded the science of dental identification. In the process of establishing a dental identification there are four major steps: (1) examining the oral region, (2) preparing postmortem records, (3) securing antemortem records, (4) comparing antemortem with postmortem records.

Even in the edentulous (without natural teeth) or partially edentulous mouth it is possible, in certain cases, to make an identification based on dentures or bridgework. Where an identification cannot be established, one should not underestimate the value in determining an exclusion—that is, being able to say that this is not the body in question.

Although the dental profession per se is becoming increasingly aware of the growing uses of dental identification, there are still many dentists with little or no knowledge of *forensic odontology,* which is the international scientific name referring to the science of dentistry as it relates to the law. Yet a dentist, at any time, might suddenly be confronted with the problem of having to identify a body by the dentition. The dentist who has had no previous experience in forensic odontology, or dental identification, will probably be at a loss as to where to begin and how to proceed.

There are few training courses given in dental identification, undoubtedly because few dental instructors have had sufficient experience in the field. At the present time a short course is offered annually at the Armed Forces Institute of Pathology, Walter Reed Army Medical Center, Washington, D.C.

The objective in writing HANDBOOK FOR DENTAL IDENTIFICATION was to produce an instructive, concise manual suggesting procedures that the dental practitioner can follow if called upon to make a dental identification. This by no means constitutes a review of all the literature and operations; rather, it is intended to be a guidebook, describing practical methods that can be utilized by the dentist in private practice who, generally, does not have available to him a forensic laboratory or complex scientific equipment. Omitted, therefore, are highly sophisticated techniques—such as histological studies of teeth for age ascertainment—that are employable by the trained academician or pathologist, but not within the realm of the practicing dentist.

As in other fields of endeavor, the more proficient one becomes, the more valuable is the assistance he is able to render. The satisfaction from performing an important community service and the excitement of working with law enforcement officers are compensation to the dentist willing to become involved in forensic odontology.

Of late, members of the medical and legal professions, law enforcement officers, anthropologists and other forensic specialists have become intrigued with the contribution that can be made to their own branches by the forensic dentist. But for the most part, their knowledge of his procedures is vague, the import of his expertise may not be fully appreciated, and an understanding of the scope of his activities may be lacking.

Since the police officer, hospital pathologist, medical examiner, prosecuting and defense attorneys will be finding themselves in increasing contact with the forensic dentist, the newest member of the medicolegal team, their cognizance of the dental procedures and the applications of forensic dentistry can do much to promote professional cooperation and a mutually beneficial relationship; whereas failure to recognize the relevancy of forensic odontology results in the forfeiture of its unique contribution as a practical science. It is hoped that this book will serve not only to instruct those in the dental profession, but also to elucidate forensic odontology for those outside the dental profession who may have occasion to work directly with the forensic dentist or to utilize his findings.

As demonstrated throughout the text, the police officer working with the forensic dentist has more than a passive role. The associative duties he can perform are many and include

—recovery of evidence and human remains
—assisting in the handling of the body
—photographing the body
—setting up and dismantling equipment
—tracking down and procuring antemortem evidence
—establishing communications and relaying material and information
—providing transportation

Cases in which I was the forensic dentist have been used to illustrate actual problems that can be encountered. The Summons Data Sheet (Chapter 2) was devised to aid the dentist, when called into a case, in consolidating the information then available that is pertinent to the dental investigation. To achieve a comprehensive postmortem Dental Identification Record (Chapter 5) that would still be clear and concise, entailed careful pruning of superfluous, seldom-used material. Since the roots of the teeth are rarely the basis for an identification, they have been eliminated from the diagrammatic chart to provide more room for the common notations. Should an individual case occur where root configuration, skull formation or other infrequently used identifying factors are involved, that information can easily be noted on the record form.

Scattered references throughout the text to carting, x-raying and photography are purposely brief to avoid, as much as possible, repeating material dealt with more fully in a specific chapter. Duplicating x-rays, explained in Chapter 6, is an important technique that serves to reduce the chance of loss of, or damage to, critical evidence. Chapter 8 defines antemortem evidence (it can be other than dental records) and suggests ways of securing it. While many dentists are skilled in using a camera, others are not. That disparity is taken into consideration in the chapter that, necessarily, touches only briefly on photography as used in forensic odontology. A glossary of dental terms as used herein and additional cases in forensic odontology are contained in the Appendix.

I wish to express appreciation to Dr. Leonard F. Menczer, Dental Director, City of Hartford; Major Benjamin Goldstein, Assistant Director, Connecticut Planning Committee on Criminal Administration; and Major George J. Fagan, Commander of Staff Services, Connecticut State Police, for reading the manuscript and offering suggestions. I also wish to thank Sergeant Richard G. Chapman, Director of Photography, Connecticut State Bureau of Identification, and his staff and Mr. Richard J. Wolfe, Rare Books Librarian, Countway Library, Harvard Medical School, for their assistance.

In conclusion, an accolade should go to the Connecticut State Police for being the first agency to have implemented in their Bureau of Identification a program in forensic odontology, which I was privileged to set up in 1960. It has given me a unique opportunity to acquire, from the hundreds of cases in which I participated as the forensic odontologist, insight and data relevant to the development of total procedures involved in assembling an unbroken chain of evidence upon which to base dental identification.

Hartford, Connecticut — LESTER L. LUNTZ, D.D.S.

Contents

Handbook for

Dental Identification

Techniques in Forensic Dentistry

1 Historical Introduction To Dental Identification

Forensic dentistry (or forensic odontology, which is the international name) refers to the science of dentistry as it relates to the law and has several phases. It may involve (1) claims seeking compensation for dental injury, (2) dental malpractice, (3) dental fraud and (4) identification by means of the dentition. The last phase is the one that concerns us in this Handbook, namely, dentistry pertaining to investigations conducted by the medical examiner's office and law enforcement agencies.

This application of dental knowledge is not limited to modern times. History records instances of identity having been determined through a superficial observation of the oral cavity and the teeth. Probably the earliest recorded incident of dental identification by a dentist dates back to the eighteenth century, when a dentist recognized in the mouth of the deceased the prosthesis that he had constructed.

FORERUNNER OF FORENSIC ODONTOLOGY

Paul Revere (Fig. 1-1) had already earned a reputation as a copperplate engraver and accomplished silversmith when he opened an office in 1768 for the practice of dentistry. His dental techniques had been learned from John Baker, an English surgeon dentist who had practiced briefly in Boston.[1]

1. Forbes, E.: *Paul Revere & the World He Lived In*, Sentry ed., pp. 129–130, Boston, Houghton Mifflin Co., 1942.

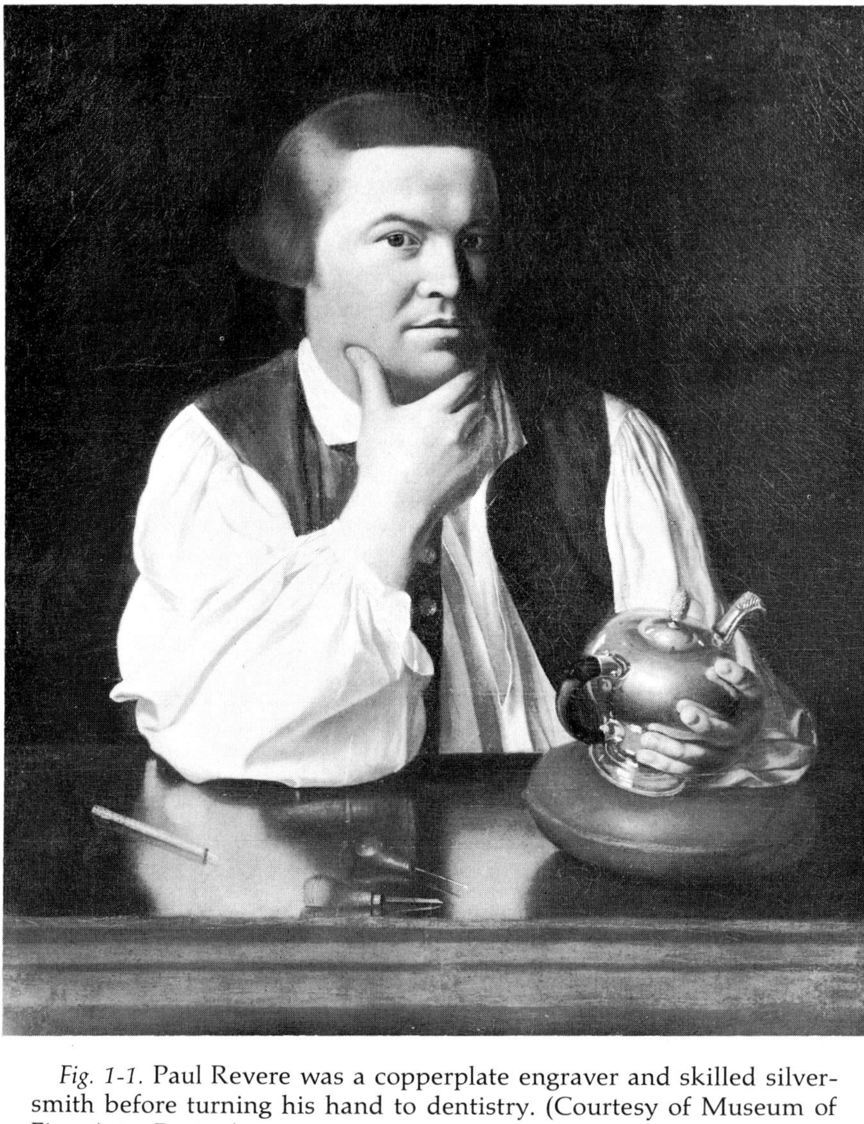

Fig. 1-1. Paul Revere was a copperplate engraver and skilled silversmith before turning his hand to dentistry. (Courtesy of Museum of Fine Arts, Boston)

Shortly before the Battle of Lexington in 1775, Revere constructed for a close friend, Dr. Joseph Warren (Fig. 1-2), a silver wire fixed bridge containing a cuspid that was probably made from hippopotamus tusk, a material then commonly used for artificial teeth.[2] Warren, a graduate of Harvard and scion of a distinguished family;

2. Ibid., pp. 131 and 477.

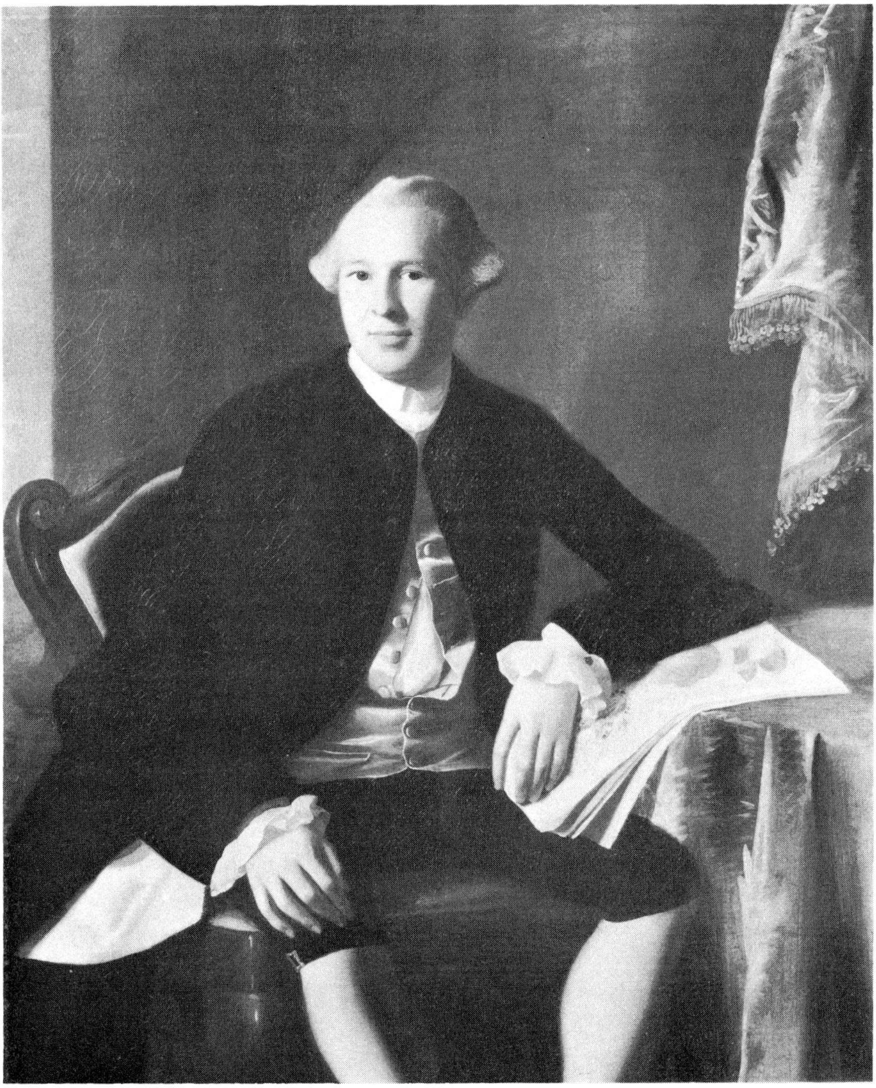

Fig. 1-2. Dr. Joseph Warren, Major General, Massachusetts Militia. (Courtesy of Museum of Fine Arts, Boston)

a leader of the Sons of Liberty, which advocated the overthrow of the British Crown; Grand Master of the Masons, and one of the instigators of the Boston Tea Party, sent his dentist friend on a famous ride to alert the militia and warn the countryside that the British were coming.

Although a major general, Warren declined to take command in

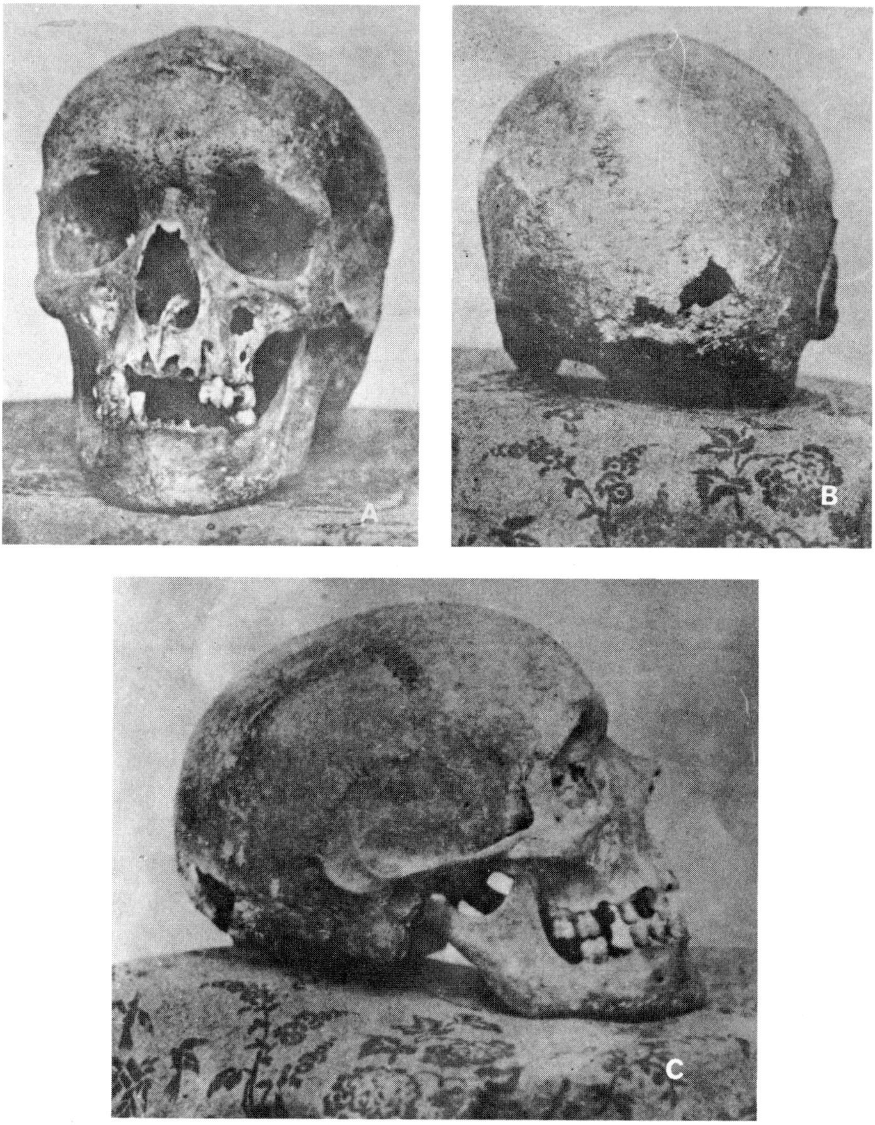

Fig. 1-3. Three views of the skull of Joseph Warren, taken by Author (L.L.L.) from a composite print made when Warren was again exhumed in 1855. Original print was traced by the Author to the sub-basement of Old South Meeting House, Boston. *A,* Fatal bullet entered skull above apex of second bicuspid on upper left side in the region of the canine fossa. *B,* Posterior view of skull, showing exit hole of bullet. *C,* Right lateral view of skull.

the Battle on Breed's Hill (erroneously referred to as the Battle of Bunker Hill), choosing, instead, to serve in the ranks with the men. There he died, at the age of thirty-four, killed instantly by a bullet that pierced his cheek and exited through the back of his head (Fig. 1-3).

Buried by the British, he was dug up the next day and reburied in a shallow grave with another American reportedly clothed in a "farmer's frock".[3] Warren's body was stripped, and his fine, expensive clothing hawked by a British soldier.

Ten months later, brothers and friends of Joseph Warren, including Revere, crossed over the Charles River to the bottom of Breed's Hill, seeking to recover Warren's body. At the gravesite they uncovered two corpses—one in a farmer's frock and the other, whom they believed to be Warren, lying unclothed. Revere confirmed the identification by recognizing in the mouth the silver wire bridgework that he had constructed for Warren a year before. General Joseph Warren was given a hero's burial on April 8, 1776.

THE CRITICAL DENTAL EVIDENCE IN THE WEBSTER-PARKMAN MURDER CASE

The province of forensic dentistry in court proceedings does not encompass the determination of guilt or innocence, nor does the dentist, in the role of expert witness, have the prerogative to encroach upon any areas of legality. His participation is limited to an attempt to establish identity through professional evaluation of the dental evidence. The case of the Commonwealth of Massachusetts against Dr. Webster in 1850 marks a milestone in dental-judiciary history, since it is probably the earliest recorded court case in which dental evidence was used to prove the corpus delicti.

Dr. John White Webster (Fig. 1-4), Professor of Chemistry and Mineralogy at Harvard Medical School, was frequently in financial straits, unable to support his extravagant tastes and a predilection for high living on a salary of less than $2,000 a year. Having expended the inheritance from his father, a wealthy apothecary, Webster commenced, in 1842, a series of loans from his friend, Dr. George Parkman (Fig. 1-5), physician and graduate of Harvard Medical School, who had become a moneylender and administrator of con-

3. Ibid., p. 315.

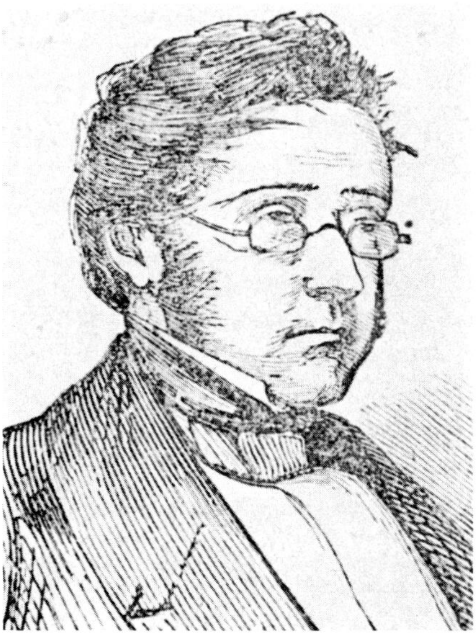

Fig. 1-4. Dr. John White Webster, affable participator in the social and cultural life of Boston, was hard pressed to maintain a proclivity for self-indulgence on the modest annual stipend that he received at Harvard.

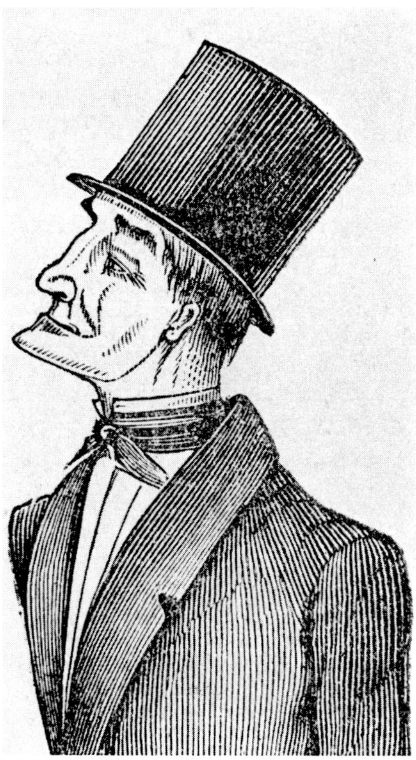

Fig. 1-5. Dr. George Parkman, wealthy benefactor of Harvard Medical School, had forsaken the medical arts in order to manage his many real estate holdings.

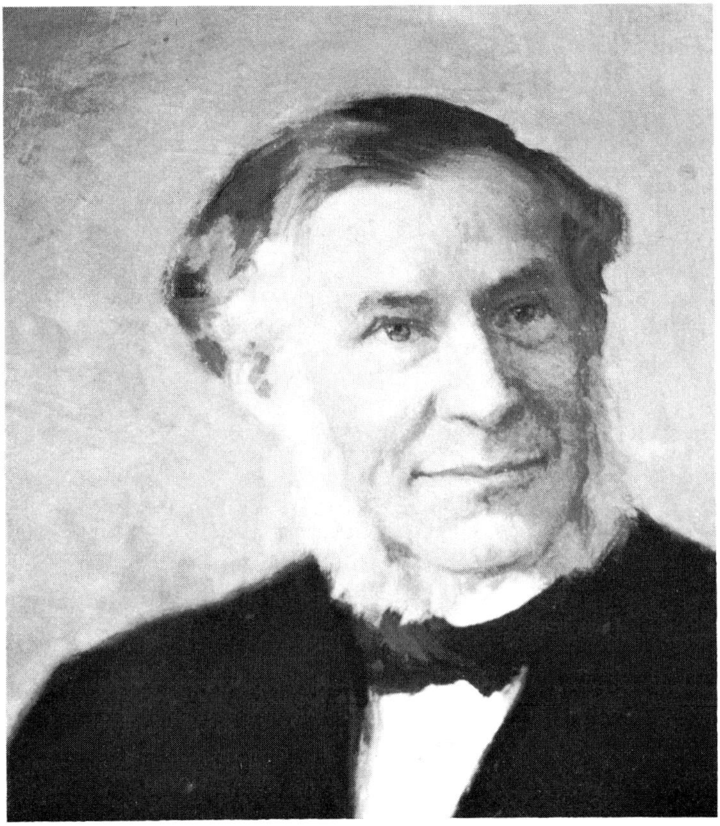

Fig. 1-6. Dr. Nathan Cooley Keep, who later became first dean of Harvard Dental School, used mineral (porcelain) teeth of his own manufacture and design when constructing dentures for Dr. Parkman in 1846. (From a painting in Harvard School of Dental Medicine)

siderable inherited property. The eccentric Dr. Parkman was a familiar sight to Boston—his prominent lower jaw thrust forward as he strode briskly about (he seldom traveled by carriage), regularly collecting his rents.

In 1846 Parkman approached Dr. Nathan Cooley Keep (Fig. 1-6), an eminent Boston dentist, about a new set of dentures. Harvard was planning to dedicate to Parkman a new medical school building constructed on land that he had donated. Although little time remained for the fabrication of the dentures, Parkman demanded that they be ready in time for the dedication ceremony.

Dr. Keep, who had been Parkman's family dentist since 1825, worked assiduously to comply. The day before Parkman's appointment, an accident occurred in the firing of the porcelain, forcing Keep and his assistant to labor through the night in order to have the dentures completed. They were inserted into Parkman's mouth just thirty minutes before commencement of the dedication ceremony.

Dr. Webster continued borrowing money from Dr. Parkman. By 1847 he owed Parkman $2,432 and had assigned his valuable mineral collection as security for the last loan.

Finding himself further embroiled in debt, Webster approached Robert Gould Shaw, Jr., brother-in-law of Parkman, for a loan of money, volunteering the same gem collection as collateral. Shortly thereafter, in conversation, Shaw mentioned to Parkman that Webster, needing money, had offered him his mineral collection.

Infuriated by the duplicity, Parkman paid Webster a hasty visit, accusing him of fraud and threatening exposure. He also began to harass Webster for repayment of the debts. Hoping to amend matters and appease Parkman, Webster suggested that Parkman meet him in his office, located next to the dissecting room in the medical building. The punctilious Dr. Parkman was seen on Friday, November 23, 1849, shortly after noon, ostensibly on his way to the medical school. He never returned home.

A week later, the dismembered remains of a body were discovered in the privy in Webster's office by the ingratiating janitor, who also found pieces of a porcelain denture and crushed skull in the furnace in Webster's laboratory. When Dr. John Webster was charged with the murder of Dr. George Parkman, all Boston was aghast.

Public preoccupation with the trial that ensued was heightened by the prominence of the leading characters. So intense was the interest generated that spectators in the gallery were permitted only ten minutes in the crowded courtroom before having to relinquish their places to others waiting outside.

On the witness stand, Dr. Nathan Cooley Keep, upon being shown the charred teeth and pieces of porcelain denture that had been removed from the furnace, identified them as the dentures he had constructed for Dr. Parkman in 1846.

> The most perfect portion that remained was *that* [italics] block, that belonged to the lower left jaw. I recognized the shape and the outline, as being identical with the impression left on my mind, of those that

> I had labored on so long. . . . On comparing the most perfect block with the model, the resemblance was so striking, that I could no longer have any doubt that they were his.[4]

Describing the manner in which he had taken impressions of Parkman's mouth, Dr. Keep exhibited to the Court the original models (Fig. 1-7) from which the dentures had been made, calling attention to the similarities between the models and the blocks that had been recovered from the furnace (Fig. 1-8). Remarking on the peculiarities of Parkman's mouth—the excessively protruding lower jaw combined with an underdeveloped upper jaw—Keep recalled that the complexity of the case and the limited time allowed for its completion had required that he and his assistant exercise constant, meticulous care.

Thereafter, Keep continued to see Parkman, on occasion, to make minor adjustments in the dentures. One evening, two weeks before his disappearance, Dr. Parkman came unexpectedly to the home of Dr. Keep, seeking to have the spring on his dentures repaired. Although it was after ten o'clock and Keep, not feeling well, had retired for the night, he dressed and came downstairs. Keep spent half an hour repairing the spring and checking the dentures to be sure everything else was satisfactory. That was the last time Dr. Keep saw Dr. Parkman professionally, although he did speak briefly with Parkman on another matter the day before he disappeared and, at that time, noticed the dentures in Parkman's mouth.

Continuing his testimony, Keep explained that porcelain dentures, because of their porosity, absorb saliva. Consequently, had the porcelain dentures been suddenly placed in direct contact with the heat of the furnace they would have exploded. That this had not occurred supported the contention that the head had been committed to the furnace with the dentures retained in the mouth and thereby shielded from the heat, so that the moisture was drawn off slowly. Moreover, under direct heat the springs in the dentures would have snapped, causing the upper and lower dentures to separate. The fact that they were together when found further indicated that they were within the head of the victim when he was relegated to the furnace.

Keep's assistant at the time, Dr. Lester Noble, testified that he

4. Bemis, G.: *Report of the Case of John W. Webster,* Boston, Little, Brown and Co., 1850.

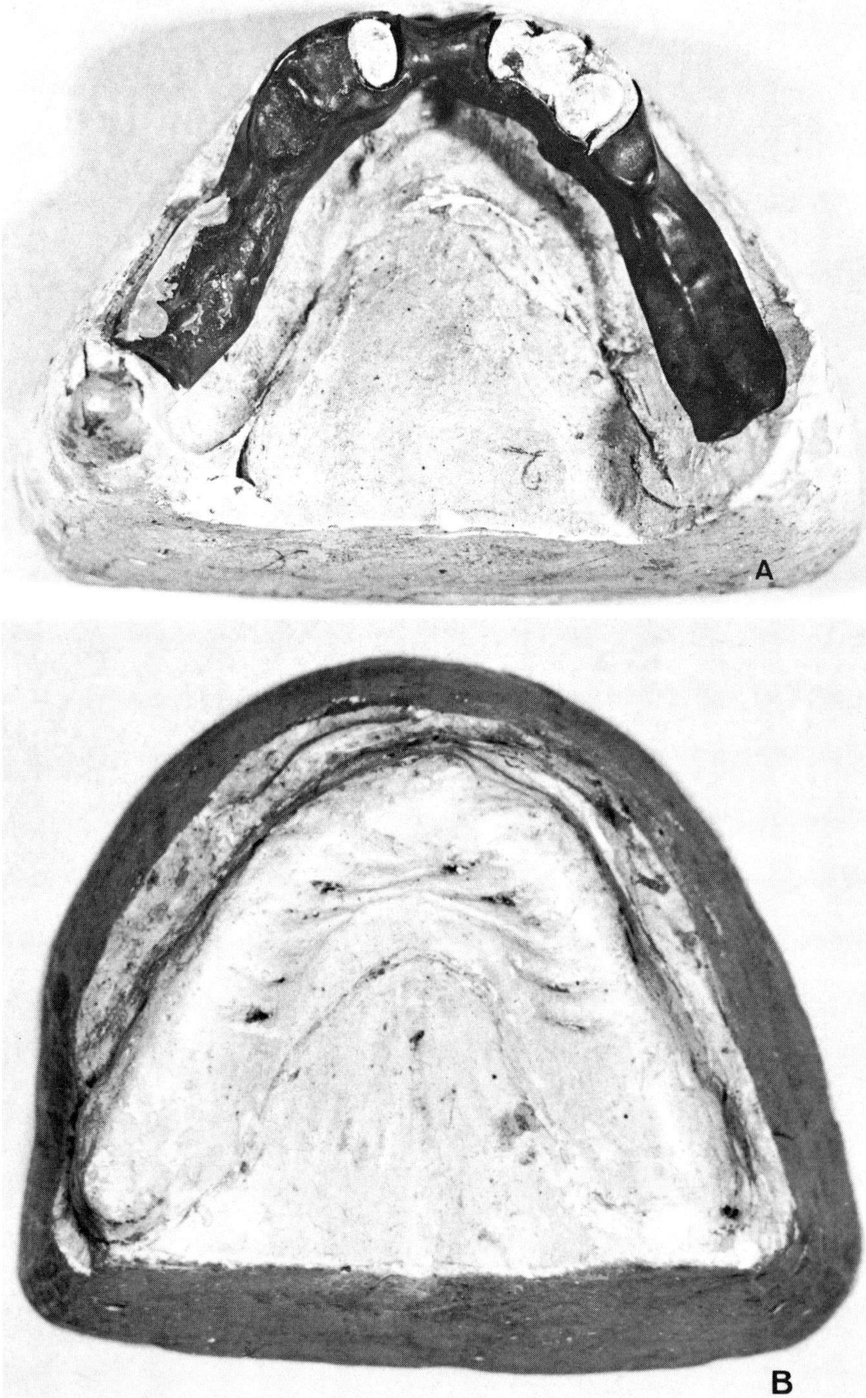

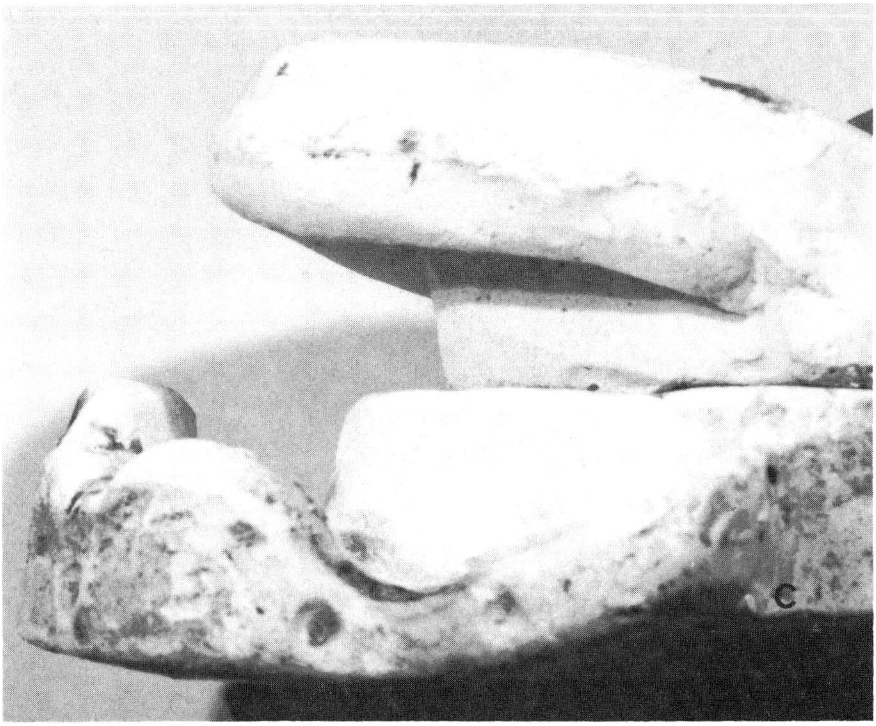

Fig. 1-7. Photographs taken by Author (L.L.L.) show the actual plaster models and wax carvings made of Dr. Parkman's mouth by Dr. Nathan C. Keep in 1846. Donated by Keep in 1867 to the Harvard Dental School Museum, the models and wax-ups are now ensconced in the Francis A. Countway Library of Medicine, Boston. There is no record of what happened to the parts of the dentures exhibited at the trial. Most of Keep's denture techniques are not used today.

A, Model of lower jaw with copper trial plate in position. The trial plate was used to check the accuracy of the model. If the trial plate fit the mouth satisfactorily, plate gold, which would form the base of the denture, was then cut and swaged. Observe interstices in trial plate that accommodated the natural teeth remaining in Parkman's lower jaw. *B,* Maxillary model of Parkman's mouth, showing distinct reproduction of rugae (raised folds on anterior palate of maxilla). Rugae, like fingerprints, are unique to the individual and are recognized as a modern technique for identification. *C,* Articulated models. The extreme loss of alveolar bone in the lower left posterior was noted by Keep in his testimony. Also evident are the protruding mandible and underdeveloped maxilla that characterized Parkman's physiognomy.

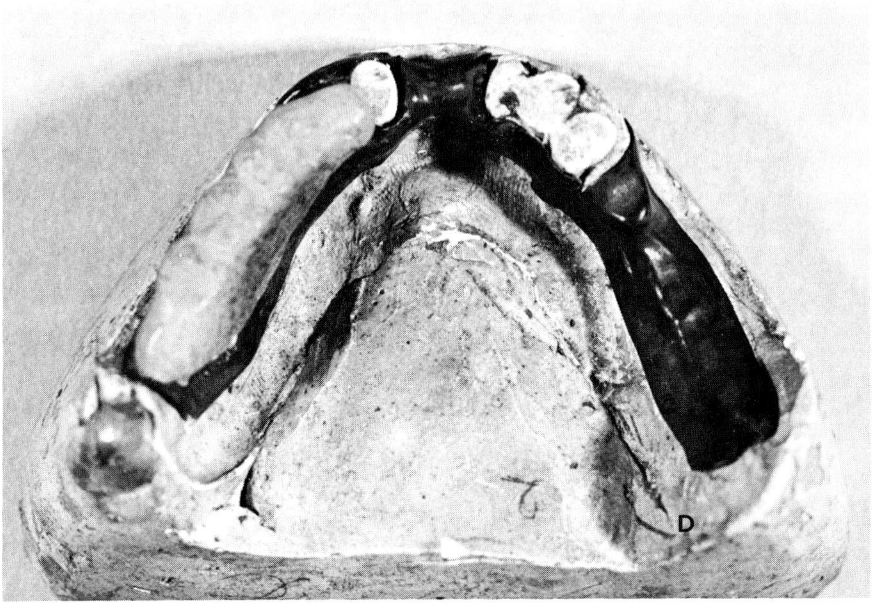

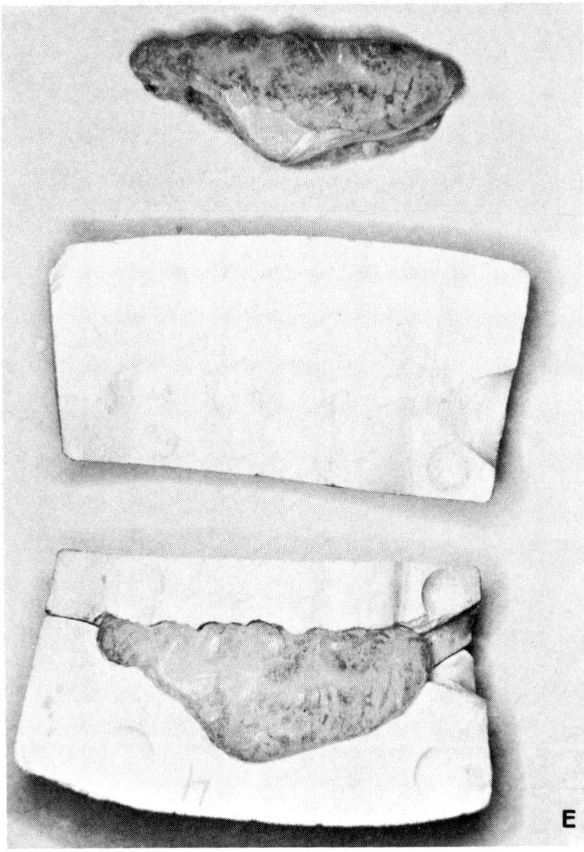

Fig. 1-7. D, Mandibular model with copper trial plate in position. On left side is wax-up of denture gum and teeth. *E,* Two wax carvings of left section of mandibular denture, made from the articulated model. They matched the largest and best-preserved section of porcelain denture recovered from the furnace in Webster's office and identified by Dr. Keep as part of the denture that he had constructed for Dr. Parkman. Bottom wax-up is set in the original plaster matrix.

himself had written Parkman's name and the date, "Oct., 1846," into the mold previously shown the Court by Dr. Keep. Dr. Noble, stating that he clearly recalled the circumstances of the case, confirmed, unequivocally, that these porcelain remains were the teeth that he and Dr. Keep had made for Parkman.

The defense, seeking to discredit the dental evidence, called to the stand Dr. William T. G. Morton, physician and dentist, distinguished for his innovative use of ether in dental surgery. Morton considered it unlikely that a dental practitioner would be able to remember the appearance of a specific denture constructed over two years before. While conceding that a dentist might recollect a particularly unusual case, where the jaw was peculiarly shaped and the denture was made fairly recently, he denied that the prominence of Parkman's jaw was unique. Morton further opined that although an entire denture made for one person would probably not fit another, portions of it might.

No direct eye witnesses to the crime were produced. When the judge in his charge to the jury stated that the salvaged bones alone were inconclusive evidence on which to resolve the case, it became the responsibility of the jury to decide the credibility of the dental evidence used to establish the corpus delicti.

Dr. Webster was found guilty of murder and sentenced to death. After an unsuccessful appeal for mercy, he was hanged August 30, 1850.

Almost a century and a quarter later, there are some who, upon reviewing the impassioned spectacle of Webster's trial, experience the uneasy feeling that justice may not have been served. In a time far removed from the attendant emotions, they are inclined to question not only the conduct of the case but also the role enacted by the janitor. Despite its debatable resolution, the case, notwithstanding, remains monumental in legal and dental history.

Since these two landmarks in forensic dentistry, there have been innumerable instances, involving single and multiple victims, where dentistry was the critical determinant in identification. In modern times especially, the value of dental identification is rapidly being recognized, and its utilization by law enforcement agencies is proliferating. With continuing progress in dental knowledge augmenting the techniques at his disposal, the forensic dentist can expect to play an expanding role in the science of identification, contributing his expertise whenever he is called upon to participate as a member of the medicolegal team.

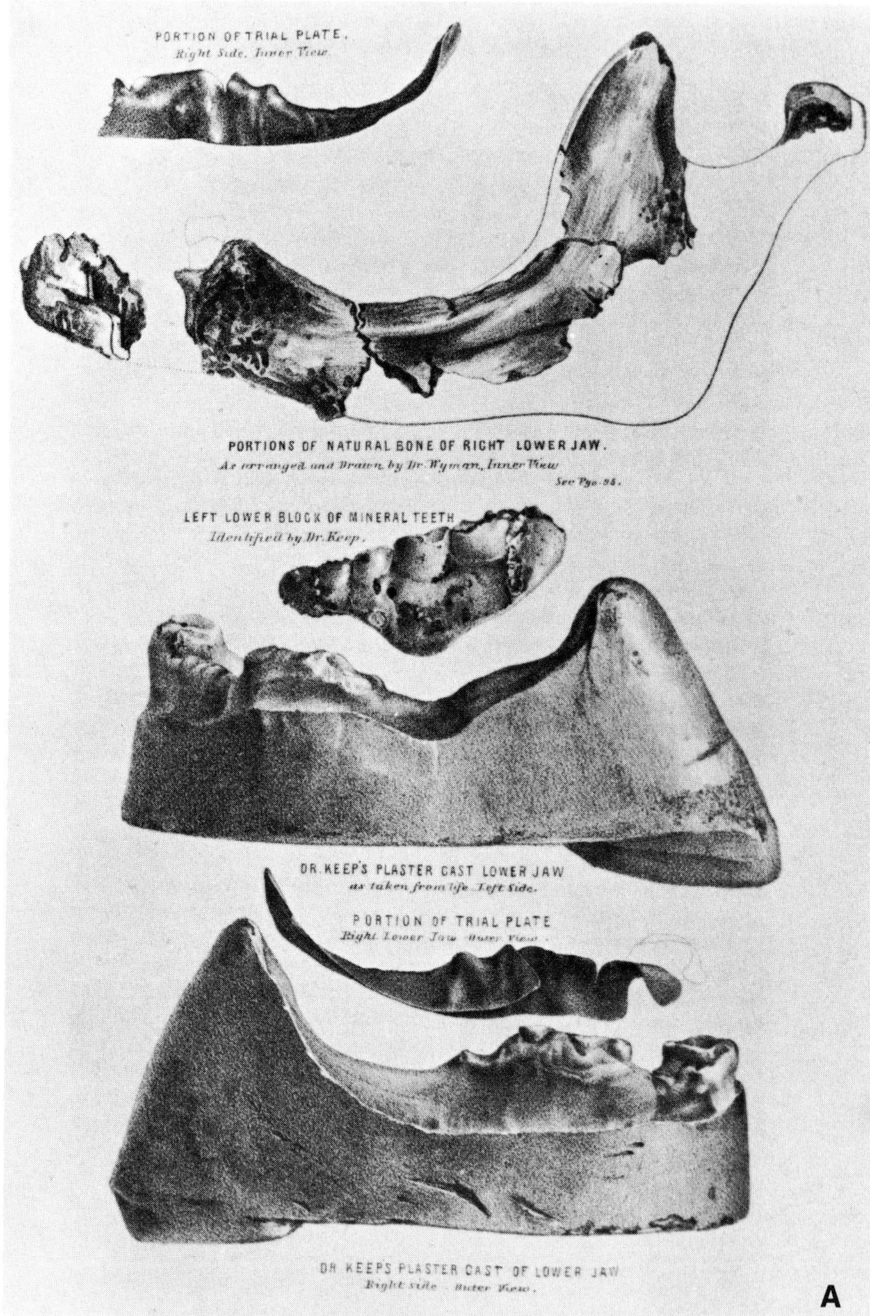
PORTION OF TRIAL PLATE.
Right Side, Inner View.
PORTIONS OF NATURAL BONE OF RIGHT LOWER JAW.
As arranged and Drawn by Dr. Wyman, Inner View
LEFT LOWER BLOCK OF MINERAL TEETH
Identified by Dr. Keep.
DR. KEEP'S PLASTER CAST LOWER JAW
as taken from life. Left Side.
PORTION OF TRIAL PLATE
Right Lower Jaw
DR KEEPS PLASTER CAST OF LOWER JAW
Right side
A

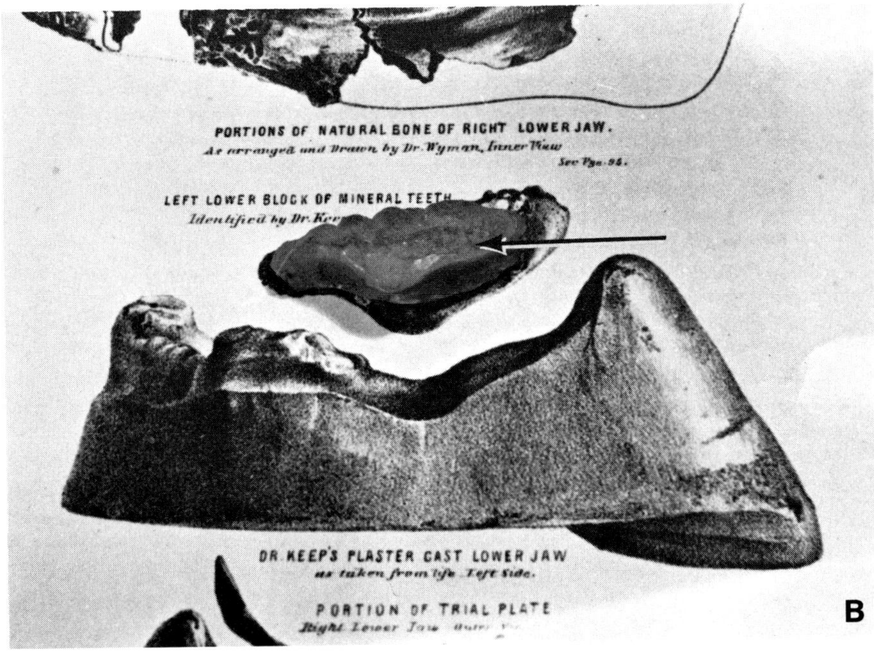

Fig. 1-8. A, Wyman's drawings (Dr. Jeffries Wyman, Professor of Anatomy at Harvard Medical School) of the dental evidence, made at the time of the Webster trial. Photography in that period was in its infancy, and drawings were commonly used. The left lower block of mineral teeth recovered from Webster's furnace (*center*) appears to fit the plaster cast of Parkman's jaw (*directly below*). Note loss of alveolar bone depicted in the drawing and evident in the articulated models in Fig. 1-7*C*. *B,* Wax-up (*arrow*) of lower left section of denture (see Fig. 1-7*E*) superimposed by Author on Wyman's drawing of the mineral teeth that were recovered from the oven. Note similarities.

2 The Summons

Dental identification should be employed only after other methods of identification have, for one reason or another, been deemed unsuccessful or inconclusive. If it is possible to determine identity visually or through fingerprints or body markings, such as scars and tattoos, then the dentist should not be summoned. Duplication of effort and needless waste of professional time are to be avoided, and that should be impressed upon police officers working in the field of identification.

When all other techniques of identification have been exhausted and it appears that the particular skill of the forensic dentist is needed, he will probably be summoned by the police or medical examiner's office. If there is no forensic dentist on their staff, the selection of a dentist may be somewhat haphazard. He may be the dentist of the person presumed to be the deceased or, merely, a local dentist known or referred to one of the investigators.

Most commonly it will be a telephone call to the dentist, requesting his assistance in identifying a body, that initiates the dental proceedings. It behooves the dentist, upon entering the case, to ascertain certain facts, recording them on the Summons Data Sheet (Fig. 2-1).

Fig. 2-1. The Summons Data Sheet (SDS) is a compilation of facts pertaining to the dental investigative proceedings. Generally, the information recorded will have been acquired through telephone communication, especially at the time the forensic dentist is initially contacted by the medical examiner's office or law enforcement agency. Since the forensic dentist is constantly on call, it is suggested that he keep SDS blanks available both in his office and at home.

DENTAL IDENTIFICATION SUMMONS DATA SHEET

1. Date ______________ Time of call ______________

2. Name of caller ______________ Rank ________ Badge No. ________

   Police Department ______________________________

   Calling from ______________________________
   address

   Can be reached at ______________________________
   address

   Telephone ______________ Extension ______________

   Name of senior investigating officer ______________________

3. Cause of death (if known) ______________________________

4. Where body found and under what circumstances ______________

   ____

5. Condition of body ______________________________
   normal, decomposed, burned, mutilated

6. Police Case No. ____________ Medical Examiner's No. ____________

   Name of medical examiner ______________ Telephone ____________

7. Present location of body ______________________________
   name of hospital, morgue, mortuary, etc.

   Address ____

   Person holding body ______________________________
   name position

   Telephone ______________ Extension ______________

8. If body is distant, can skull or jaws be brought locally for the dental examination? ______ When? ______________

   Dental examination to be performed at ______________________
   name of hospital, mortuary, etc.

   Address ____

   Best route to site of dental examination ______________________

   ____

   ____

   ____

over

9. Missing person who might be the deceased:

Name____________________ Age______ Race____________________

Address____

10. Dentists who have treated missing person:

Dr.____

Office address____

Home address____

Office telephone____________ Home telephone________________

Dr.____

Office address____

Home address____

Office telephone________________ Home telephone____________

11. Have antemortem records been secured?_____ List______________

12. Persons who might have information to aid identification:

Name______________________ Telephone__________________

Address____

Relationship to deceased________________________________

Name______________________ Telephone__________________

Address____

Relationship to deceased________________________________

13. Assisting police officers:

Name______________________ Department_________________

Name______________________ Department_________________

14. Other data____

____

____

____

At the outset he should be assured that all other techniques of identification have been exhausted, and therefore, the services of a dentist are required in an attempt to obtain an identification by means of the dentition. He should inquire the identity and authority of the person telephoning him. If it is a police officer, note his name, rank, badge number and department, also the locale of the call and the telephone number and address where he can be reached should it be necessary to speak to him again. If he is not the senior officer in charge of the investigation, inquire who is.

Other pertinent data include the cause of death, if known, police case number and medical examiner's number, present location of the body (name of hospital, funeral parlor, morgue, etc. and the address) as well as the name, position and telephone number of the person holding the body. The dentist should also inquire whether there has been speculation as to the possible identity of the deceased. If a person has been reported missing who might be the deceased, ask the name, address and telephone number of the next of kin and of the dentist who has treated the missing person (if that information has been obtained), and whether antemortem dental records are available.

Moreover, knowing the condition of the body (usually burned, mutilated, decomposed, a combination of these, or normal) can aid the forensic dentist by helping to prepare him mentally and emotionally for the task at hand. The dentist should receive the permission of the medical examiner to perform the necessary procedures.

If the body is a considerable distance away, the forensic dentist might ask about the feasibility of having a pathologist or mortician resect and prepare the skull or jaws, depending upon the condition of the body, to be brought locally for the examination (Figs. 2-2 and 2-3). That accommodation not only would conserve valuable time for the dentist but also would permit him to operate in more familiar surroundings. If it is not possible, he should request explicit directions as to the best route there. The person holding the body should be apprised of the name and arrival time of the dentist, and his cooperation should be solicited.

The forensic dentist should request from the investigating police department the assistance of one or two officers, preferably from the Identification Bureau and at least one who is capable of using a press-type camera. Besides photographing the body, the police officer would witness the dental procedures and could record them on film.

A competent police officer, under the direction of the dentist, can

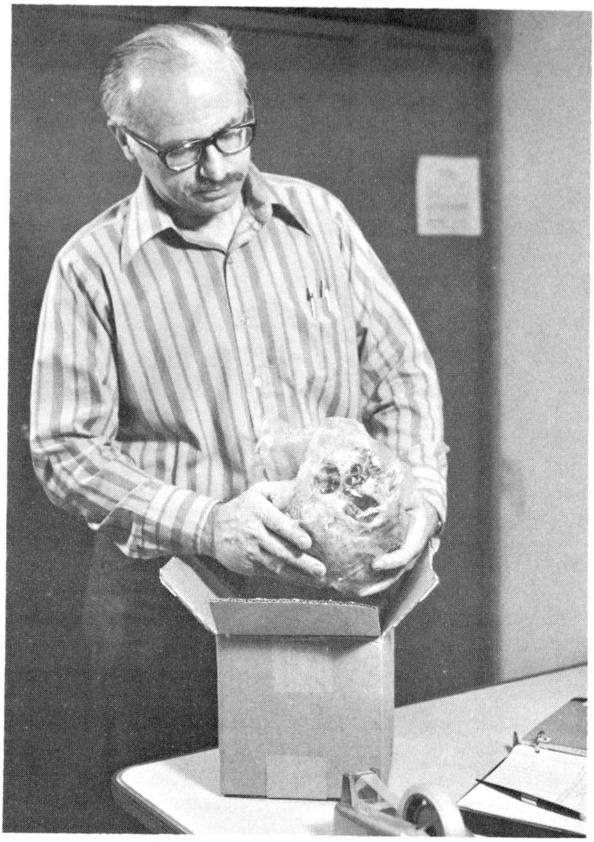

Fig. 2-2. The skull or resected jaws must be properly packaged if they are to be relocated for the dental examination. Where the body has been decapitated or is completely decomposed, it is not difficult to carefully package the whole skull. A polyethelene bag, since it is airtight, makes an excellent wrapper for dry specimens, which are then put into a box or other suitable container for transport. However, should any flesh remain on the skull or resected jaws, it might require that they first be placed in preservative solution and then securely boxed.

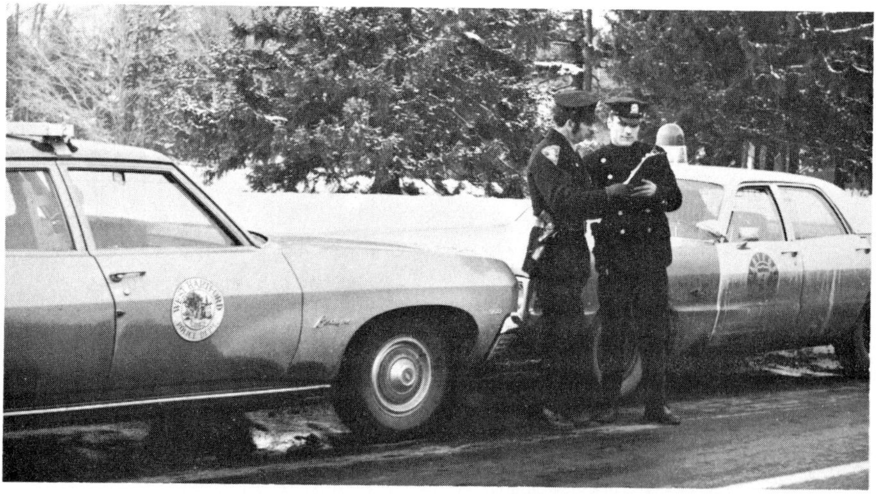

Fig. 2-3. Skull, jaws, records, etc. can be transported quickly by police, in relays if necessary. Receipts should be signed at transferral points to facilitate tracing, should the need arise.

aid in many ways, thereby enabling the dentist to operate more efficiently and speedily. The officer can assemble and disassemble instruments and equipment, assist in charting the mouth, serve as ancillary during the performance of some of the surgical procedures and, in some cases, assume the responsibility for obtaining antemortem records. The dentist, if not provided with police transportation, should arrange to have the assisting police officers meet him at the location of the body.

During the course of the telephone call, all transcribed information should be repeated and the names of persons and places spelled to insure accuracy. Depending upon the information the dentist has been given, he may attempt, before proceeding to the case, to locate dental antemortem records. It is desirable to have the antemortem records on hand at the time of the dental examination, but not always possible, and occasionally considerable sleuthing is required in order to track them down. To facilitate the search for dental records, the forensic dentist should have at his disposal a directory of the dentists registered to practice in the state, obtainable from the State Dental Commission. A comprehensive directory of dentists is also published by the American Dental Association.*

When there are multiple victims in a case, it is usually advisable to use a Summons Data Sheet for each. The Summons Data Sheet should be taken to the examination and updated, where indicated, as the dental investigation proceeds. Thus, the Summons Data Sheet serves as a source of reference pertaining to the dental aspects of the case and, if properly maintained, will guide the dentist not only in his preparation and approach to the examination but in the search for antemortem records as well.

*American Dental Association, 211 E. Chicago Avenue, Chicago, Illinois 60611.

3 The Dental Identification Kit

The instruments and equipment contained in a dental identification kit differ from those used routinely in a dental office, being requisite to the particular procedures in dental identification. Because the forensic dentist is constantly on call, not knowing when his services may be needed, it is advisable that the special armamentarium be retained intact, readily accessible and in good operating condition. On concluding a dental examination, the dentist should resterilize the instruments and make any necessary replenishments, so that the kit will be in order for the next assignment.

Because each case is different and has its own special problems, it is impossible to predict precisely what the dentist will encounter as he commences a dental investigation—the specific conditions under which he will have to operate, the facilities that will be available, the amount of assistance that he will receive or other contingencies. He should strive to be as self-sufficient as possible, taking the complete armarium to each case so as not to find himself in the situation of needing an item that he neglected to bring.

If the work of identification is to be performed in a funeral home, he would not expect most instruments or equipment to be available. However, where the forensic dentist will be working in a hospital morgue, it is likely that he will be operating under optimal conditions and that the instruments and equipment he requires will be placed at his disposal. By taking advantage of such opportunities, he can spare his own paraphernalia.

Some police departments are better equipped than others, administratively and materially, to assist the dentist, while many, having had little, if any, previous experience with dental identification, may be ignorant of his needs or the manner in which they can aid. Ideally, a police agency or medical examiner's office would maintain a well-equipped dental identification kit. Funds for this might come from city, county, state or Federal sources or from private grants.

Factors to consider in assembling a kit are weight, portability, fragility, cost and convenience. Including as many disposables as possible lessens the need for washing and sterilizing, the convenience outweighing any possible cost factor. Most of the instruments and equipment can be obtained from a dental or medical supply company. In the following list, wherever it seems expedient a manufacturer's name is given with the idea that this may facilitate procuring the item. Similar items, equally acceptable, may be produced by other manufacturers, but understandably, it is impossible to mention them all. Throughout the text, where price is stated, it is intended to be merely a guide and is, necessarily, an approximation.

THE CARRYING CASE

The instruments and equipment used by the forensic dentist, with the exception of camera and x-ray equipment, can be entirely contained in a portable case measuring approximately 21 × 14 × 7 inches (Fig. 3-1). It should have hard sides, a durable handle and be sturdy enough to withstand the jolting of a car and all the use to which it will be subjected. Whether there is a key lock is a matter of choice, the disadvantage lying in the chance of losing, misplacing or simply forgetting to take along the key. Suffice it to say that neither the container nor its contents should be left where they could easily be stolen.

A suitable case might be found in a luggage shop or surplus store. With ingenuity, a man's valise could be adapted, any inner dividers or pockets being utilized advantageously to effect an orderly storage of the contents. A metal case, like that used for a portable typewriter, also might make a satisfactory container.

Dental and medical instruments to be carried inside the kit should first be wrapped in a sectioned, canvas instrument roll, such as the Army uses, which is sometimes sold in surplus stores. To include cameras and x-ray equipment in the carrying case along with the other items would make it unduly cumbersome. Furthermore, because of their fragility, cameras and portable x-ray equipment should

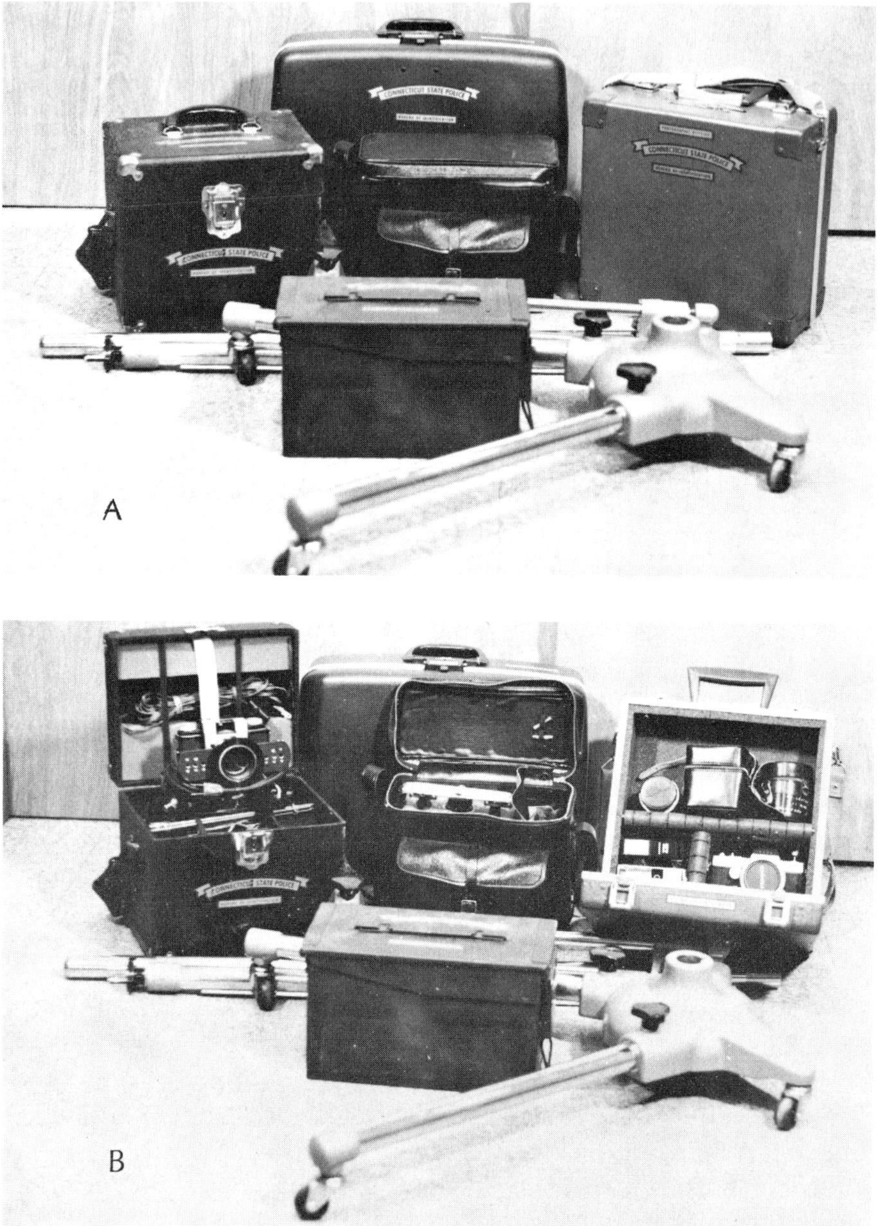

Fig. 3-1. Cases holding armarium used in dental identification. *A,* (*Rear*) Dental identification kit (inside are instruments, tape recorder, face masks and other supplies); (*center, left to right*) case with dental camera rig, camera-type case with portable x-ray equipment (x-ray machine, timer cord, AC cord, x-ray film and film holders), camera case with additional photographic gear; (*front*) Army ammunition case containing portable x-ray developing equipment (Uni-Chem set and ruby bulb) and (*right*) unassembled mobile stand for x-ray machine. *B,* Open cases display armamentarium.

be carried separately in their own special cases and always carefully placed where they are not liable to fall or be broken.

The name of the forensic dentist and the agency with which he is associated (i.e., police or medical examiner's office) should be plainly marked on the exterior of the cases. Where practicable, an identifying mark on the individual items themselves would minimize the possibility of mix-up with equipment belonging to the premises where the dentist is working. An electric metal engraving tool can be used on the stainless steel instruments, while other items can be labeled with a Dymo tapewriter.

INSTRUMENTS, EQUIPMENT AND OTHER SUPPLIES

A well-equipped dental identification kit will include all of the items mentioned below. Of course, if cost is not a limiting factor, additional items, while not absolutely necessary, can contribute to the ease and efficiency with which the dentist works. The skull chisel, for example, is an effective instrument, used by pathologists, to pry apart sectioned bone. A dentist who does not possess that instrument, however, might have access to it when working in the autopsy room of a hospital. The quantities suggested below will suffice for the usual dental identification case, taking into account that the forensic dentist will wish to provide aprons, cotton rolls, face masks, gloves, etc. for the use and protection of those who may be aiding him. A mass disaster, obviously, will necessitate increasing supplies accordingly.

Dental Mouth Mirrors. Include at least 5 mouth mirrors, No. 5, plane (not concave), front surface (the reflecting surface is processed on the front of the mirror, eliminating the distortion present when the reflection comes from within a thickness of glass). The dental mouth mirror (Fig. 3-2) is used for retraction, reflection of light and reflection of the area of the mouth under examination. The nondisposable ($3.15 apiece) is sturdier than the disposable ($7.50 per hundred) and for that reason may be preferred.

Dental Explorers. Straight-handled, stainless steel instruments, single- or double-end, with sharp points, explorers are used for examining the pits and fissures of teeth and the margins of restorations (Fig. 3-3). Include single-end Nos. 6, 17 and 23 ($2 apiece) or double-end Nos. 1 and 5 ($3 apiece). That selection, having the angulation of

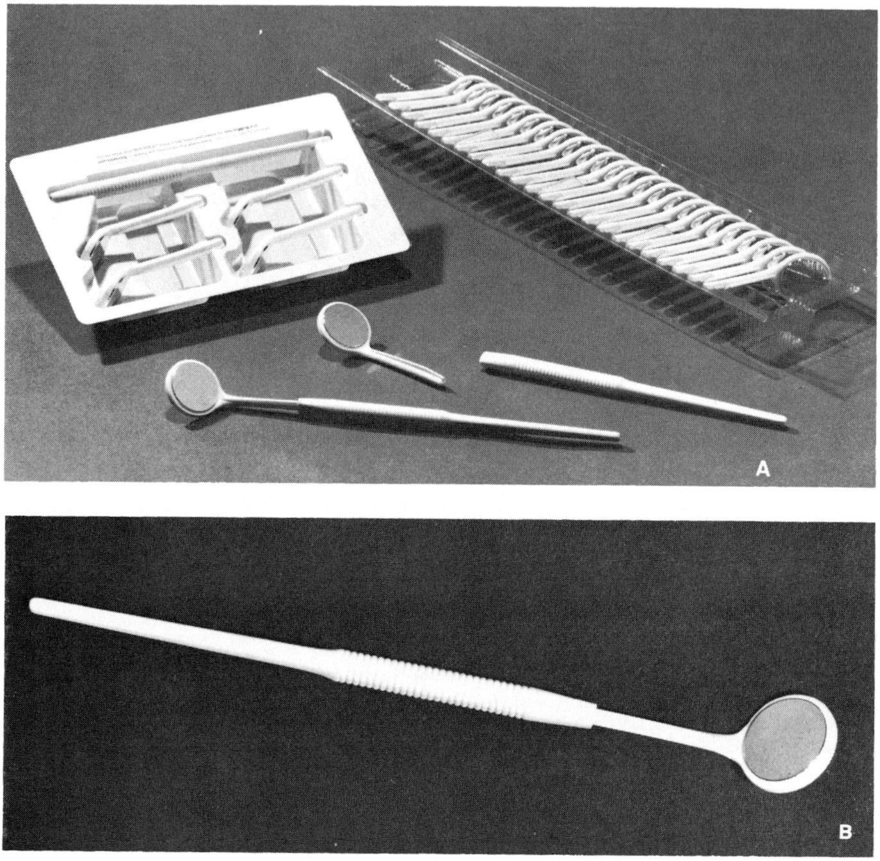

Fig. 3-2. A, Disposable front surface mouth mirror. The same handle can be used repeatedly; the mirror head is replaced after each usage. *B,* Close-up of Belvac disposable mouth mirror. (Photographs courtesy of Belvac International Industries, Ltd.)

the pointed tip in different relationships to the handle, enables the examiner to get into most locations in the human mouth.

Molt Mouth Prop. The Molt mouth prop ($30) is designed to force and hold the mouth open (Fig. 3-3).

Scalpels. Scalpels are surgical knives used for cutting soft tissue (Fig. 3-4). Because the blades tend to break in heavy use, keep on hand at least 5 disposable scalpels with No. 20 blade ($2.90 per box of ten).

Hemostats. Hemostats are useful for retracting and holding tissue

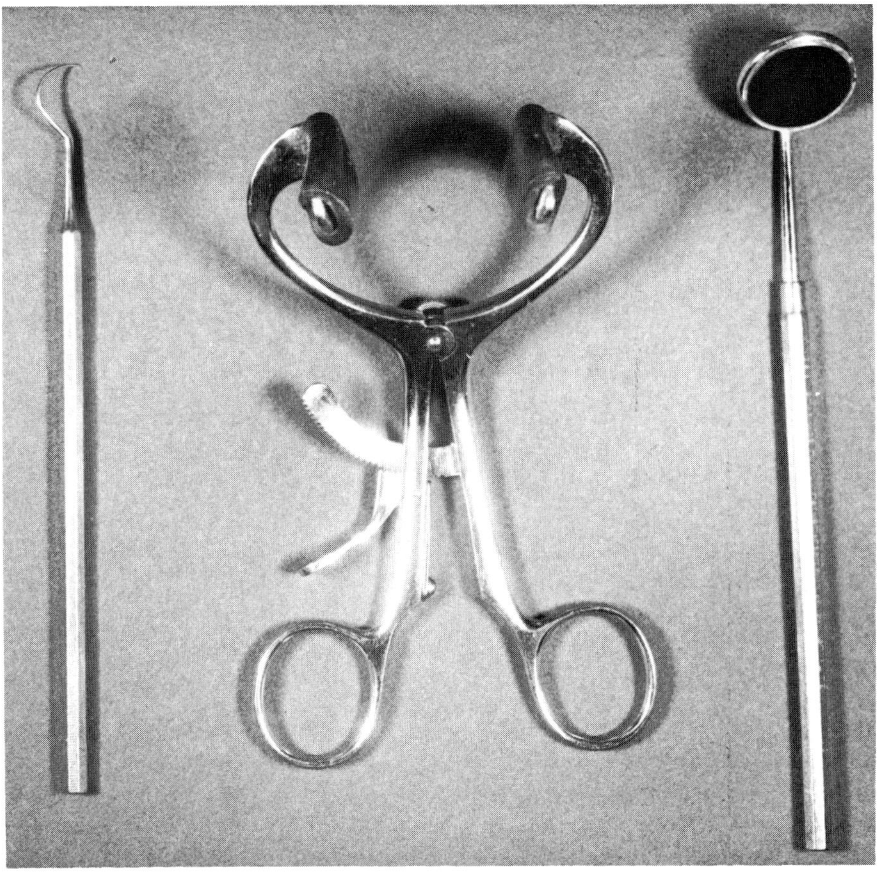

Fig. 3-3. (*Left to right*) A No. 23 single-end, stainless steel, dental explorer; Molt mouth prop; and stainless steel, front surface dental mouth mirror.

(Fig. 3-4). Include one $6\frac{1}{2}$-inch straight ($7.50) and one $6\frac{1}{2}$-inch curved ($7.95), both nondisposable.

Surgical Scissors. For cutting tissue include one $5\frac{1}{2}$-inch scissors with straight blades and, preferably, sharp points ($9) and one $5\frac{1}{2}$-inch scissors with curved blades (Fig. 3-4) and sharp points ($9.20).

Surgical Bone Saw. Used for cutting bone, the surgical bone saw ($22.50) is operated manually. If the budget is greatly restricted, an ordinary hardware hacksaw or keyhole saw can substitute.

Headlight. The headlamp ($55), consisting of a light attached to a headband, enables the dentist to spotlight the area that he is exam-

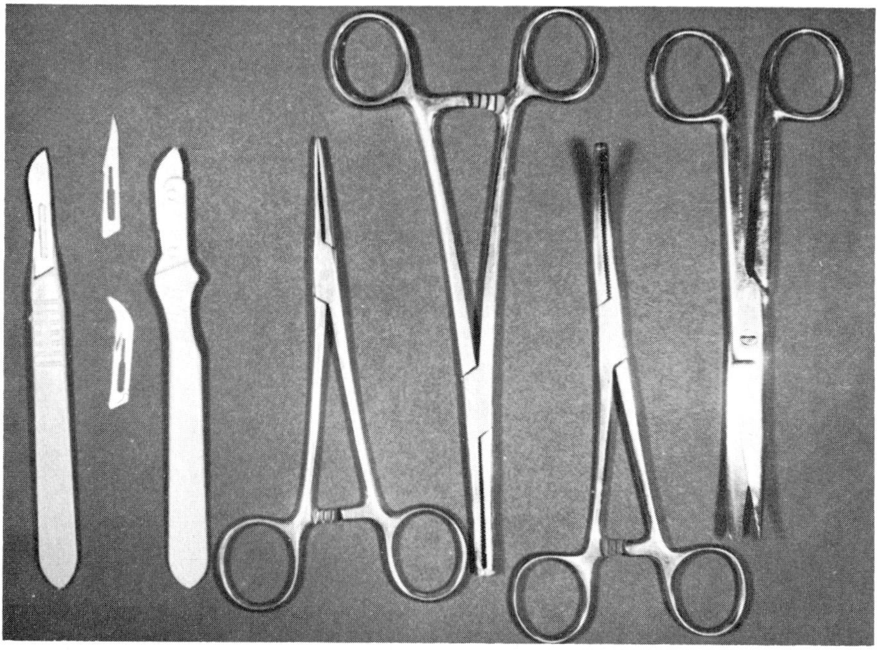

Fig. 3-4. (*Left to right*) Disposable scalpel that can be used with interchangeable blades, shown here with blade No. 10; two interchangeable blades, (*upper*) No. 11 and (*lower*) No. 12; disposable scalpel with blade No. 20, not interchangeable; three hemostats, two straight and one curved; and a surgical scissors with curved blades and one sharp point.

ining, still leaving his hands free. It should operate on low voltage current to decrease the possibility of electrical shock (Fig. 3-5).

Dental Diagnostic Flashlight. A penlight used for examining the mouth, the dental diagnostic flashlight ($7.50) comes equipped with interchangeable lucite heads and a dental mouth mirror (Fig. 3-5). It can usually be obtained from a dental supply house. Source of power is two AA flashlight batteries, whose vitality should be checked occasionally.

Gauze Pads and Cotton Rolls. Include one small package of 4 × 4-inch gauze squares for cleaning teeth and tissue and one package of 50, No. 2 dental cotton rolls, $1\frac{1}{2}$ inches. When required, the cotton rolls are suitable for placement in the nostrils of those present at the dental examination to shut out obnoxious odors (Fig. 3-6).

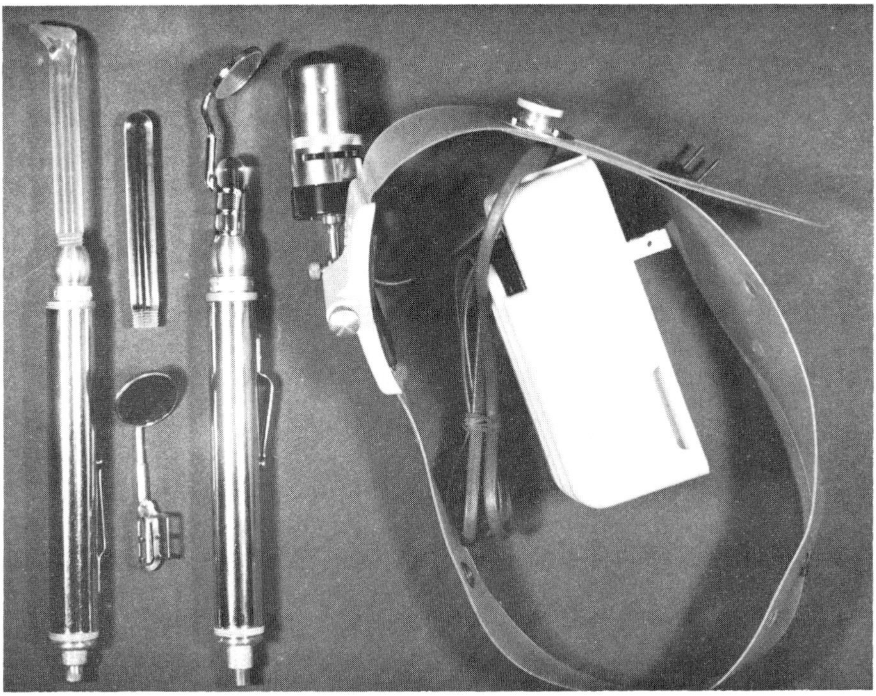

Fig. 3-5. Dental diagnostic flashlights and headlamp: (*left to right*) extended, transparent lucite tube with translucent, pedate head used for lighting and retraction; detached extended lucite tube and detached mouth mirror; diagnostic flashlight with mouth mirror attached to a short, lucite head; headlight attached to adjustable headband, shown with low voltage transformer power source.

Noxzema. When used on the protruding end of the cotton rolls and dabbed around the mouth and nostrils, Noxzema aids in screening out unpleasant odors (Fig. 3-6).

Face Masks. Several types of inexpensive, disposable face masks are available (Fig. 3-7). They aid in preventing odor inhalation by retaining the cotton rolls securely in the nostrils and, also, protect the wearer against bacteria that might be present in the corpse, such as the tubercle bacillus that continues living after the host is dead. Face masks with a nose strip conform more closely to the contour of the face and have the added advantage of tending to prevent the breath from escaping and fogging eyeglasses (3M face masks, $4.95 for twenty-five). Carry 5 in the kit.

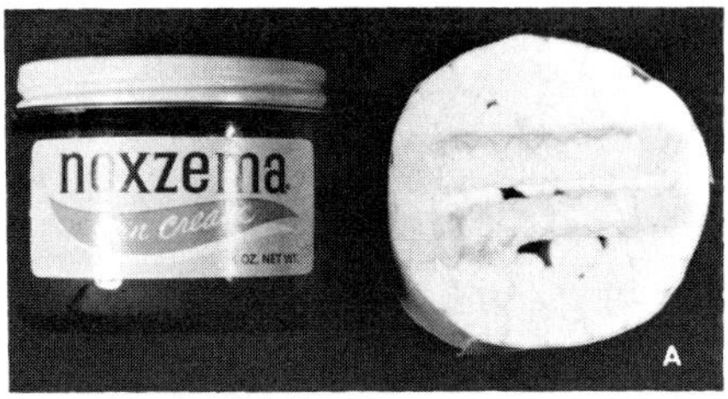

Fig. 3-6. A, Jar of Noxzema and package of No. 2, $1\frac{1}{2}$-inch dental cotton rolls, useful for screening out unpleasant, organic odors.

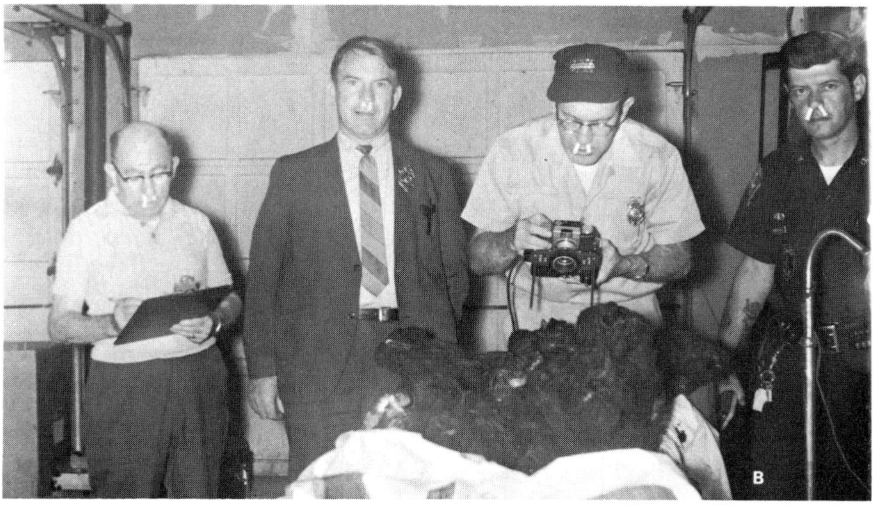

Fig. 3-6. B, Because dental cotton rolls in the nostrils obstruct normal breathing, mouth breathing is resorted to. For best results the nose should be completely packed. The scene of examination is garage of mortuary. (Glastonbury Police Department)

Willson Respirator. Recommended for less limited budgets, the Willson Respirator, Model No. 1225 ($15), permits unimpeded breathing (double filters screen out offensive, organic odors) and can be worn comfortably with eyeglasses (Fig. 3-8). It may not be regularly stocked but can probably be ordered through a medical supply company.

Disclosing Solution and Cotton Swabs. A dye disclosing solution ($\frac{1}{2}$ oz.), such as Mercurochrome, tinted benzalconium chloride or an analine dye, applied to the teeth with a cotton swab (include 5 swabs in the kit) can be used to show the margins of silicate or plastic fillings.

Rubber Gloves. Disposable latex surgeon's gloves (Fig. 3-9), 10 pairs,

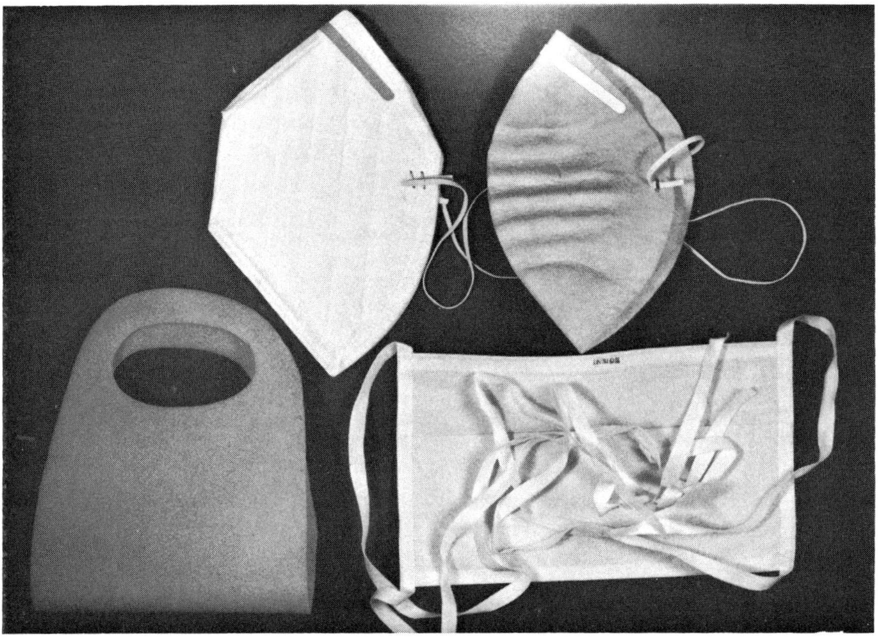

Fig. 3-7. Four different types of disposable face masks that are available commercially.

should be kept in the kit to allow for frequent changes in the event that the examiner finds it necessary to chart, photograph, x-ray and handle the body concomitantly.

Aprons. Five disposable plastic aprons are probably enough to protect the clothing of all those who come in contact with the body.

Toothbrushes. Two toothbrushes, preferably denture type because the bristles are firmer and longer, should be included for removing debris from the teeth of the corpse.

Plastic Bags. Have on hand a few plastic bags as convenient receptacles for instruments that have been used and are awaiting sterilization.

Extension Cord. A 25-foot extension cord, with multiple outlets, is essential for lighting and camera equipment when the electrical outlets are not in proximity to the body. A heavy-duty 50-foot extension cord is useful on occasion but may be too bulky to be accommodated in the carrying case.

Stationery Supplies. Include 3 sharpened pencils; 3 ball point pens; 5 Summons Data Sheets (see Chapter 2); 5 postmortem dental charts

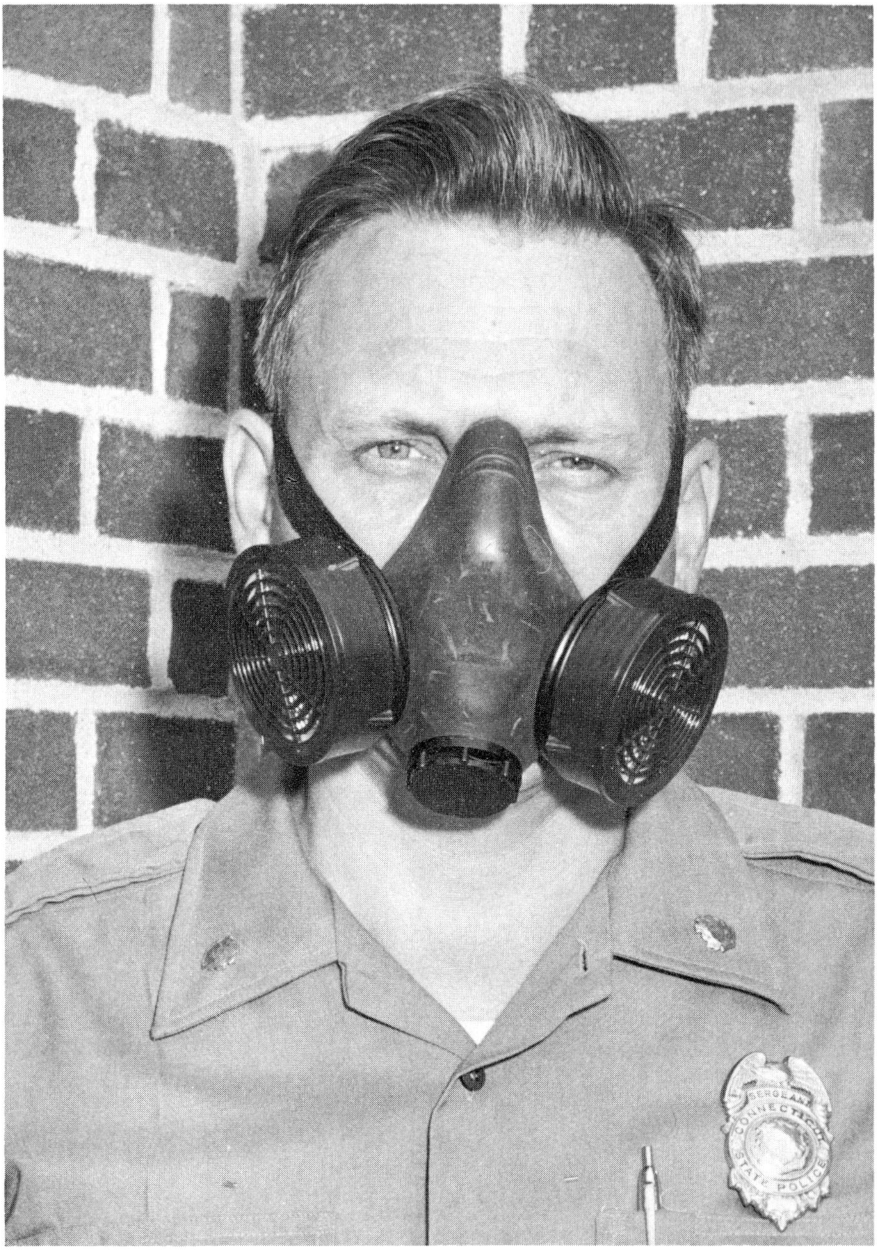

Fig. 3-8. Model No. 1225 Willson Respirator. The organic odor filtering cartridge is replaceable when it loses its effectiveness.

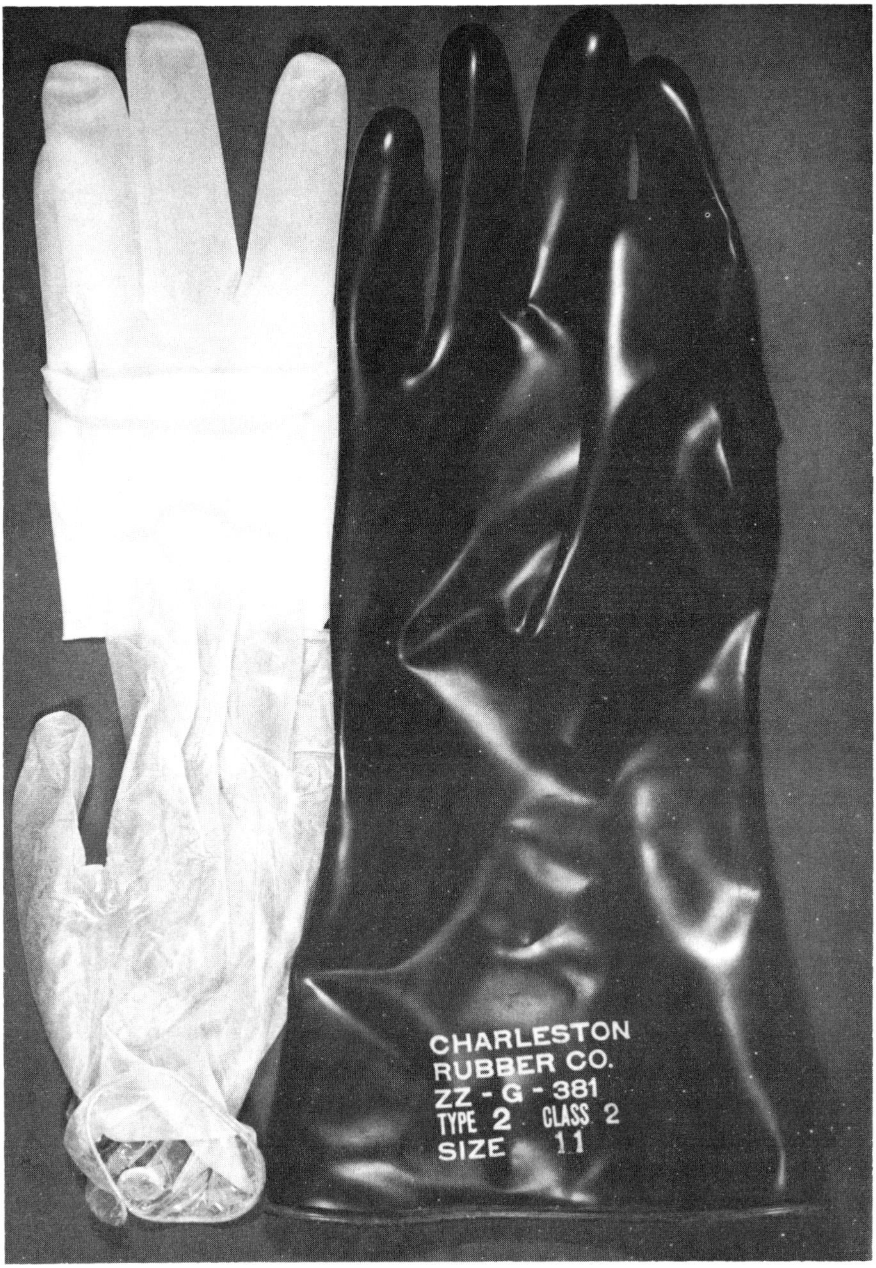

Fig. 3-9. Different types of surgeon's gloves: (*upper left*) disposable latex glove; (*lower left*) disposable thin-plastic examination glove; (*right*) heavy-duty rubber glove used by U.S. Army Graves Registration Service for body recovery in the field. The extended cuff and heavy rubber of the Army glove provide extra protection. A sturdy, waterproof, commercial household glove would be a satisfactory substitute.

(see Chapter 5); a state directory of registered dentists; 2 clipboards, one for charting and the other for the Summons Data Sheet; a metal or plastic 6-inch ruler with millimeter scale (Fig. 3-10), either can go into cold sterilization; and self-adhering millimeter measuring tapes,* useful for indicating relative size when small areas are photographed.

Tape Recorder. A verbal description of the postmortem charting can be made on a cassette tape recorder (Fig. 3-11*A*). The telephone pick-up accessory (Fig. 3-11*B*) permits the investigating dentist to record both sides of the conversation when securing summons data or antemortem information over the telephone. Cassette tape recorders vary in price (from $25 to $125), depending upon quality. The cassettes used in the recorder are self-contained, reel-to-reel cartridges (Fig. 3-11*C*), available in playing times of fifteen minutes to one hour ($1 to $5).

Photographic Equipment. Film and a camera arrangement suitable for dental photography should be included (see Chapter 7).

Stryker Autopsy Saw. A high-speed electrical saw with reciprocating action, the Stryker autopsy saw (Fig. 3-12) is faster and easier to use for cutting through bone than the manually operated surgical bone saw. However, the cost (approximately $150) may exclude it from many identification kits unless it can be purchased through a grant, gift or some other special appropriation.

Min-X-Ray. A remarkable, compact, portable x-ray machine with an output of 63–65 kilovolts and 10–15 milliamperes, the Min-X-Ray ($1500) produces good dental and medical radiographs (Fig. 3-13). It operates from any 110 to 130 volt 60 cycle AC power source or from a portable gasoline generator.† The dentist fortunate enough to possess this apparatus would include among his supplies 25 Kodak Ultra-Speed periapical films, 4 bite-wing films and a few film holders (see Chapter 6).

Uni-Chem Single Solution System. Ideally suited for use with the portable x-ray machine, the Uni-Chem Quick Tank Kit ($7.20) enables the dentist to develop his x-rays on the spot. The kit consists of an opaque, jarlike, plastic developing tank, about four inches deep and three inches in diameter; a plastic frame for holding six x-rays; and Uni-Chem solution, a single solution for developing and

*Professional Tape Company, Inc., 144 Tower Drive, Burr Ridge (Hinsdale), Illinois 60521.

† MinXray, Inc., 3535 W. Irving Park Road, Chicago, Illinois 60618.

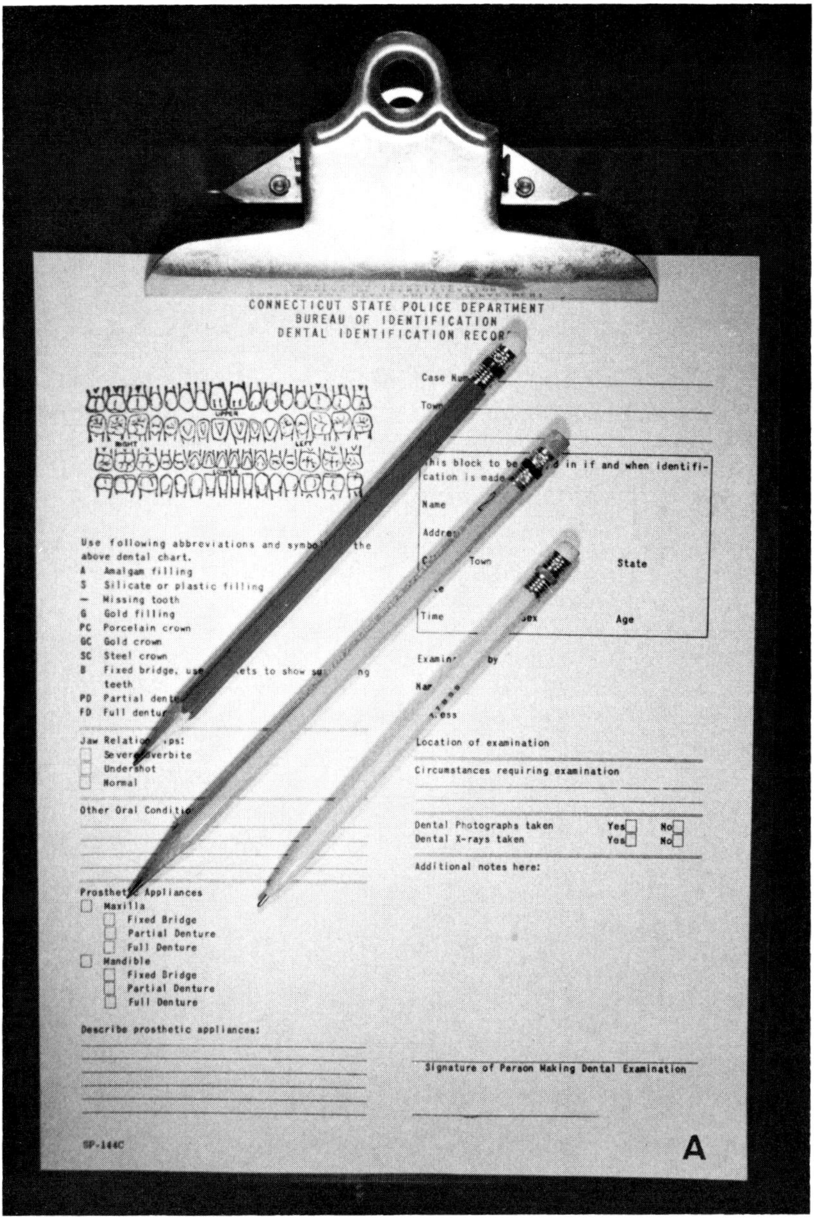

Fig. 3-10. A, Stationery supplies for postmortem dental charting include pen, pencils, clipboard and postmortem record form. It should not be assumed that pens and pencils will always be available at the scene.

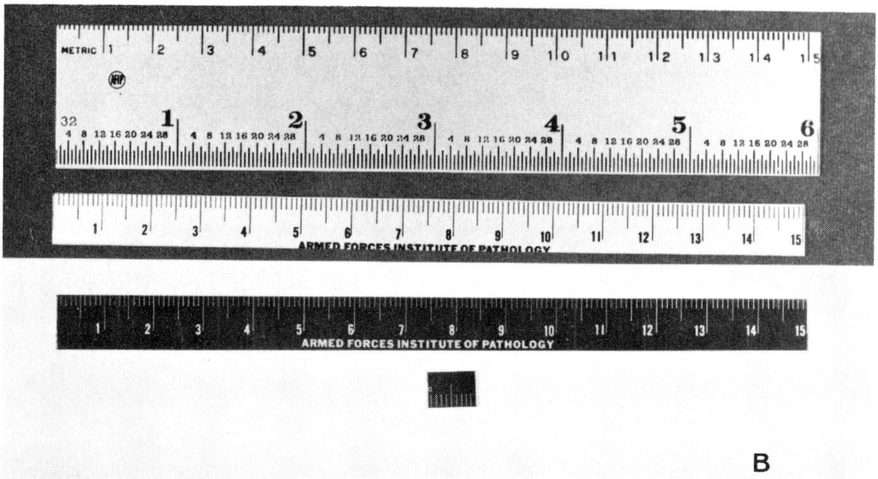

Fig. 3-10. B, Metal rulers with flat finish (nonreflecting surface), used for medical photography. White rulers are used against dark backgrounds and vice versa.

fixing only Kodak Ultra-Speed film, in three minutes at 75°F (Fig. 3-14).

Dark Room Ruby Bulb. Screwing a 25-watt 115-volt Westinghouse ruby bulb ($8 in photography stores) into an electric bulb socket in a closet transforms it into a darkroom. The problem of a closet lacking an incandescent light bulb socket is solved by utilizing the extension cord with a socket attached (Fig. 3-15).

Checklist. A checklist of instruments, equipment and other supplies (Fig. 3-16) should be kept with the dental identification kit to facilitate "checking in" the contents preparatory to the dentist's leaving for an examination and "checking out," to be sure nothing has been left behind when he is ready to depart from the scene of the investigation. Likewise, it is a handy means for taking inventory and making replenishments between assignments.

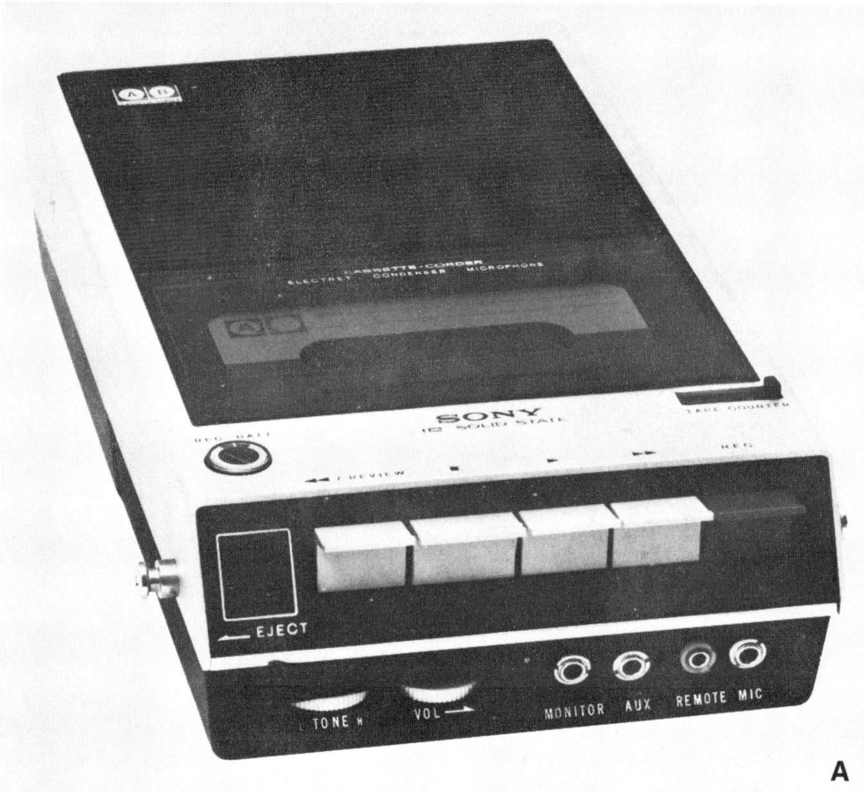

A

Fig. 3-11. A, Sony portable cassette tape recorder, Model 110A, for taping postmortem charting, antemortem information, telephone conversations, etc. Unit has a hand microphone, automatic level control and built-in microphone that can be used with foot switch to permit hands-free operation, a convenient feature at the autopsy table, since it minimizes possibility of contamination of the recorder. In addition, this model has a built-in digital counter for noting the place on the tape (Courtesy of Superscope, Inc.)

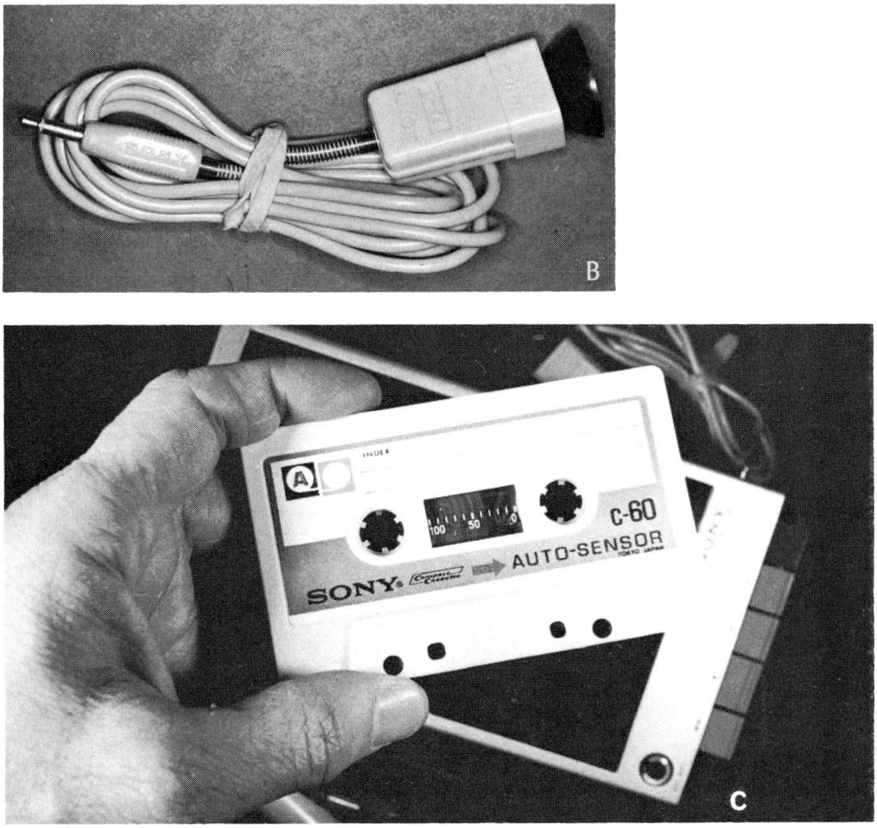

Fig. 3-11. B, The telephone pick-up accessory is an inexpensive device for recording both sides of a telephone conversation on tape. One end of the device attaches by means of a suction cup to the receiver part of the telephone handset while the other plugs into the microphone jack of the recorder. The party on the other end of the line should be informed that the conversation is being taped. Tape-recorded material can serve as a valuable, verificative adjunct to written records. *C,* The Sony C-60 cartridge, shown here, records for thirty minutes on each side. Generally, the Sony C-30 (fifteen minutes on a side) will provide ample time for charting. When used in a Sony tape recorder, the Sony auto-sensor cartridge gives an audible signal to indicate the end of the tape.

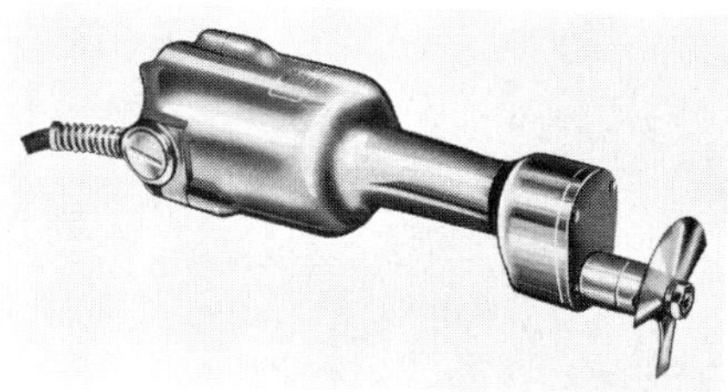

Fig. 3-12. The Stryker electric autopsy saw, Model 8209–21 with blade No. 1100, cuts bone by high-speed oscillation, facilitating resection of maxilla and mandible. (Courtesy of Stryker Corporation)

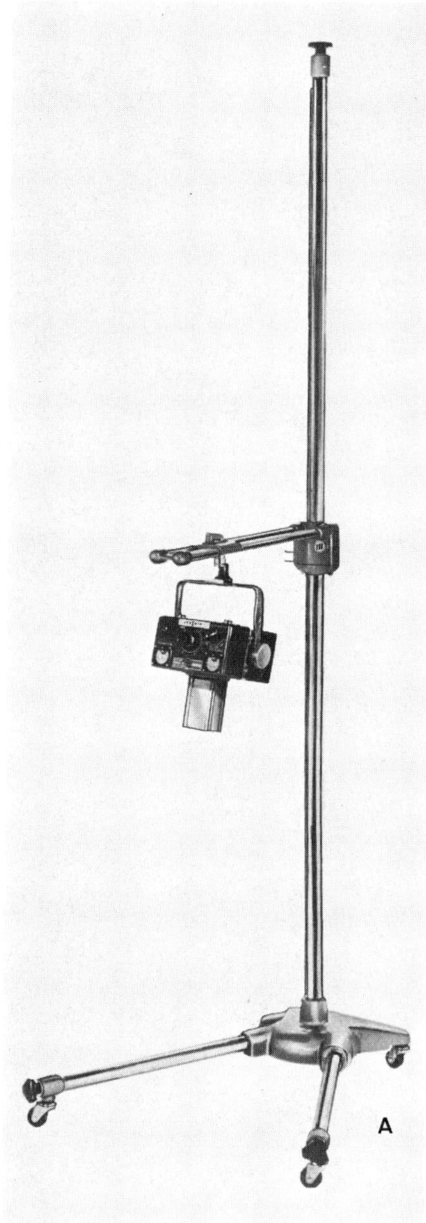

Fig. 3-13. The Min-X-Ray is a unique, lightweight, portable x-ray machine that produces good medical and dental roentgenograms with minimal scatter radiation. Easily manipulated, it comes equipped with a mobile stand, carrying case and medical or dental cone, the head and cone together weighing only 17 pounds. The Min-X-Ray can also be utilized in law enforcement work to x-ray questioned boxes for lethal explosives. *A,* Min-X-Ray machine with dental cone. (Courtesy of MinXray, Inc.)

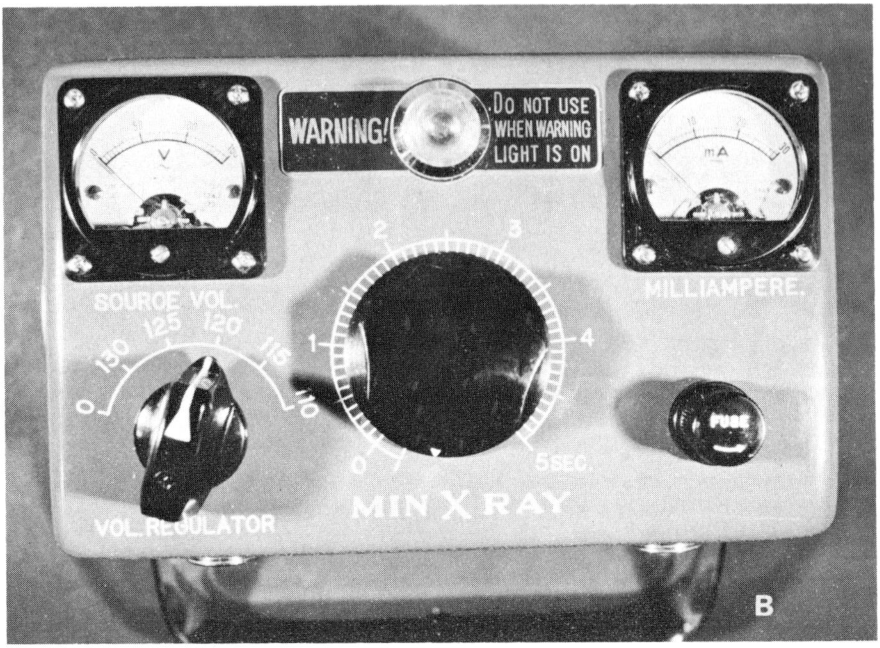

Fig. 3-13. B, Head (generator) measures $6\frac{1}{2} \times 4 \times 6\frac{3}{4}$ inches and weighs about $16\frac{1}{2}$ pounds.

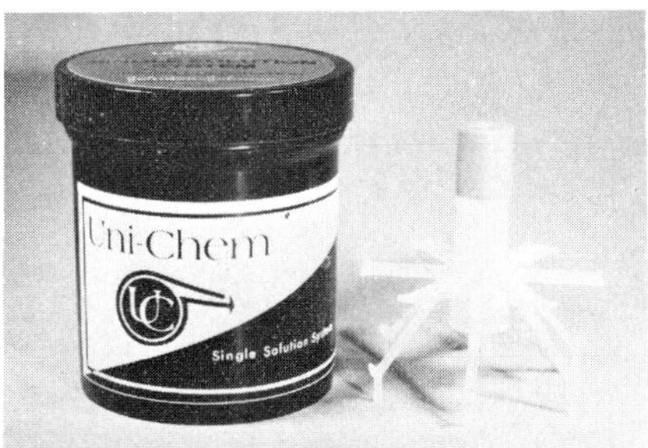

Fig. 3-14. The Uni-Chem Quick Tank Kit uses a single solution developing system that enables x-rays to be developed at the scene of an examination. Plastic frame holds six periapical x-rays.

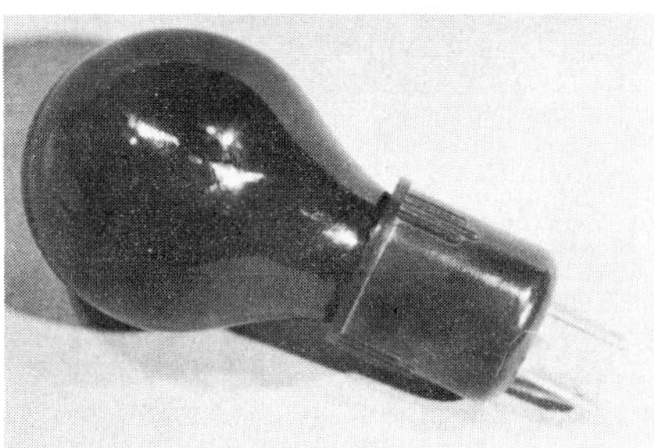

Fig. 3-15. Ruby bulb, shown here with socket attached, provides controlled lighting for developing dental x-rays at the site of an examination.

DENTAL IDENTIFICATION KIT

Checklist

	Quantity	Description
Dental Mouth Mirrors	5	plane, front surface, No. 5
Dental Explorers	3	single-end Nos. 6, 17 and 23 or
	2	double-end Nos. 1 and 5
Molt Mouth Prop	1	
Scalpels	5	disposable No. 20 blade
Hemostats	1	straight $6\frac{1}{2}$-inch
	1	curved $6\frac{1}{2}$-inch
Surgical Scissors	1	straight $5\frac{1}{2}$-inch, sharp points
	1	curved $5\frac{1}{2}$-inch, sharp points
Surgical Bone Saw	1	
or Stryker Autopsy Saw	1	
Headlight	1	
Dental Diagnostic Flashlight	1	
Gauze Pads	1	small package of 4 × 4-inch
Dye Disclosing Solution	$\frac{1}{2}$	ounce
Cotton Swabs	5	
Cotton Rolls	1	package of 50 No. 2, $1\frac{1}{2}$-inch
Noxzema	1	small jar
Face Masks	5	disposable
Willson Respirator	1	
Rubber Gloves	10	pairs, disposable
Aprons	5	disposable
Toothbrushes	2	denture type
Plastic Bags		several
Extension Cord	1	25-foot with multiple outlets
Heavy-duty Extension Cord	1	50-foot (optional)
Tape Recorder	1	with cassette
Pens and Pencils	3	each
Clipboards	2	
Dental Identification Records	5	
Summons Data Sheets	5	
Ruler	1	6-inch with millimeter scale
Metric Scale Labels	5	
Photographic Equipment		according to choice
X-ray Machine	1	portable Min-X-Ray
X-ray Film	25	Ultra-Speed periapicals
	4	Ultra-Speed bite-wings
X-ray Film Holders		according to choice
Uni-Chem Quick Tank Kit	1	complete with solution
Ruby Bulb	1	

Fig. 3-16. Specimen checklist for a well-equipped dental identification kit. The itemized accounting will vary from one kit to another. As changes in the contents are made from time to time, matching additions or deletions should be recorded on the checklist. Bite-mark supplies have been omitted, since they are used infrequently and only in particular cases (see Chapter 9).

4 Access to the Mouth

Gaining access to the mouth of the unknown deceased is a prerequisite for examining, charting, x-raying and photographing the dentition. The condition of the head at the time of the examination will determine the procedure to be employed in attaining access to the mouth.

For the purpose of classification, the head of the deceased can, generally, be described by one of the following:

1. Head in normal condition
2. Completely decomposed head
3. Burned head
4. Mutilated head
5. Partially decomposed head

Under certain circumstances there may be a combination of conditions existing in one head, as the head that is both mutilated and burned (e.g., in an airplane crash) or the head that is both decomposed and mutilated.

HEAD IN NORMAL CONDITION

The important distinction of the head in normal condition is that it can be identified readily by sight. The corpse is still in a good state of preservation with little, or no, apparent injury to the face and jaws.

The forensic dentist is summoned after other techniques of identification have been exhausted: Although visual identification is possible, no one has reported a missing person; no clues to identity, such as personal effects, laundry marks or clothing labels, have been found on the body; there is no record of fingerprints in local, state or FBI files.

Every distinguishing characteristic that might be useful for identification should be recorded prior to burial of the body. Therefore, the teeth should be charted, x-rayed and photographed. All information thus obtained will be kept on file in the event that, subsequently, a person resembling the deceased is reported missing and dental records of the missing person are available for comparison with postmortem records.

Prior to the dental examination, so that the face will not have been disturbed, the forensic dentist and assisting police officer should take photographs of the head and face. These photographs might aid in establishing identity (see Chapter 7).

When the head is in normal condition, the dental examination of the mouth is similar to that performed on the normal, living patient. It differs, however, in the following aspects:

1. The body on the autopsy table or in a casket lacks the positional flexibility of the patient in a dental chair.

2. The autopsy room or funeral parlor is not equipped with dental examining lights. (If lighting conditions are inadequate, the dentist can wear a headlamp during the examination.)

3. In all probability, the examining dentist will not have a water and compressed air syringe, as he does at his office dental unit, to clear off debris or saliva for a better view of the teeth. Occasionally suction is available in the autopsy room, but that convenience he also must be prepared to forgo.

4. A dye solution, such as Mercurochrome, tinted benzalkonium chloride or an analine dye, carefully applied to the anterior teeth with a cotton swab acts as a disclosing solution for silicate, plastic or quartz composite fillings, which, otherwise, might be difficult to detect because of their similarity in color to the natural tooth.

5. The dentist cannot have cooperation from a deceased in positioning the head, opening the mouth, holding x-ray film, etc.

6. Gloves should be worn during the examination of the dentition to avoid the possibility of contamination. Charts, cameras, tape recorder and other items that cannot be sterilized should not be handled concomitantly with the corpse. It is desirable to have a competent assistant, such as another dentist, to make notations on

the chart and manage the equipment, under instructions from the dentist performing the examination.

Since visual identification of the normal head is possible, the body may be viewed, up to the time of burial, by relatives or friends of missing persons. Accordingly, the face should be minimally disturbed, and facial tissues should not be cut to facilitate access to the mouth. (There is also the possibility that after interment the body might be exhumed.)

If necessary, before the examination and charting are begun, the mouth should be aspirated. If no aspirator is available, 4 × 4-inch gauze sponges can be used.

The Molt mouth prop, which is designed to hold the mouth open, should be carefully placed (to avoid dislodging of loose teeth) on the opposite side from that being examined. Accordingly, place the mouth prop on the left-hand side of the mouth and, with the aid of a dental mouth mirror and an explorer, commence charting on the upper right side, proceeding toward the left as far along as possible, repeating on the lower right side. Reposition the mouth prop to the right-hand side of the mouth and complete the charting on the left side.

After the charting has been completed, x-rays should be taken and, if possible, developed at the site (it can be done while the dentist photographs the dentition) for assurance that all the desired roentgenographic information has been obtained.

Color film delineates more clearly than black-and-white the shape and material (amalgam or gold) of any restorations in the mouth. Because access to the mouth of the head in normal condition is restricted, a front surface mirror designed for oral photographs will aid in photographing the occlusal (chewing) surfaces of the teeth. **Warning:** Keep all film, including that in cameras, out of the range of x-ray radiation to avoid accidental exposure.

Case History

A black female, about 20 years of age, was found dead in a housing project in Hartford, Connecticut, at 6:00 A.M. There was no evidence of injury (Fig. 4-1).

The autopsy determined she had been dead four or five hours but failed to reveal the cause of death. Although narcotism was suspected, narcotics were not detected in the laboratory tests.

No one had been reported missing, nor was there a fingerprint

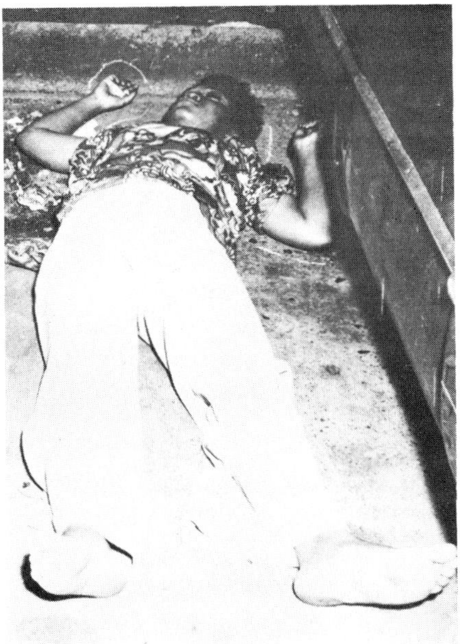

Fig. 4-1. Black female body discovered in parking lot of housing project had no signs of injury or clues to identity. The head was in normal condition, and visual identification was possible. (Hartford Police Department)

record in police files. There were no personal effects or clothing labels on the body as clues to identity.

Publication in a metropolitan newspaper of a "Wanted—Information" bulletin containing the morgue photograph (Fig. 4-2), which was deemed inoffensive for public viewing, failed to produce anyone with information about the deceased.

A dental examination revealed that the victim had two teeth missing—the lower first molars. The remaining teeth were in excellent condition, with no caries or restorations. Lateral plate x-rays were taken of each side of the deceased's mouth (Fig. 4-3) on the possibility that a dentist might have taken x-rays of the missing teeth prior to their extraction. At some future time, if a person matching the description of the deceased is reported missing and dental x-rays are available, they can be compared with the postmortem x-rays. Regrettably, up to the time of burial no identity was established, and the body was placed in a numbered grave.

COMPLETELY DECOMPOSED HEAD

Of all cases involving dental identification the completely decomposed (skeletonized) head is probably the easiest to work on. First,

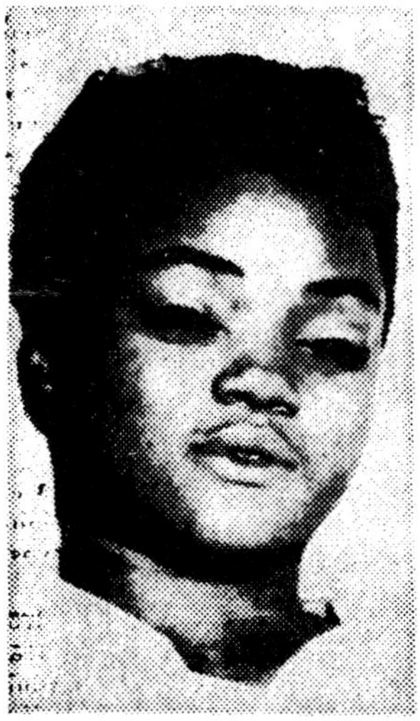

Who Is She?
Morgue Photo

Dead Girl's Identity Still Sought

Hartford Police are asking help from anyone who has information that might identify an 18-to-20-year-old girl who was found dead in a Stowe Village parking lot at 24 Kensington St., April 13.

She was found at 6 a.m. and police said she died about two or three hours earlier that Sunday morning. The cause of death had nct been determined. Police said there were no marks on the body to indicate foul play.

Fig. 4-2. Because the morgue photograph was of a normal head and not objectionable, *The Hartford Courant,* a metropolitan newspaper, was willing to publish it. However, it failed to produce any leads to identification.

there is little or no disagreeable odor. Second, because there is no tissue covering the teeth, access to the mouth is not a problem. Third, unlike jaws that have tissue encasing them, skeletonized jaws readily reveal the condition of the supporting alveolar bone. Finally, because no attachments remain, the skull is detached from the body, and the mandible, having separated from the maxilla, can be removed completely for the examination.

Care should be exercised in handling the teeth of the skeletonized head for two reasons in particular: (1) It is likely that they have dried out and are brittle; (2) Because the attachments of the teeth disintegrate rapidly after death, the teeth are readily separated from the alveoli (sockets) and, consequently, could easily be lost.

It is important, therefore, to determine whether any teeth were lost after death, and if so, a policeman should be dispatched to the area where the remains were discovered to search for teeth lost postmortem and not recovered with the body.

A tooth lost postmortem leaves a clear socket with a sharp alveolar bone margin around the edge of the socket. A socket lacking sharp margins and partially filled with bone denotes a tooth lost ante-

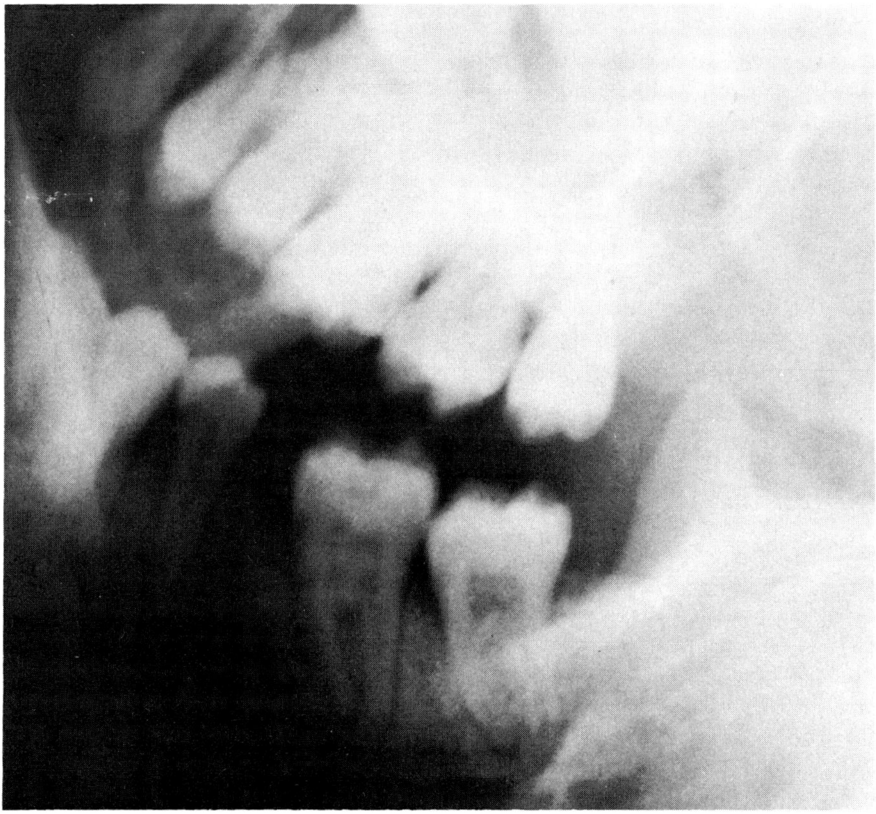

Fig. 4-3. Postmortem lateral plate x-ray shows space left by a missing molar and, also, the root formations of the approximating teeth. This x-ray can be used for comparison with an antemortem dental x-ray of the same area.

mortem; a socket completely filled with bone indicates the tooth was lost a considerable time before death—probably nine months to a year or more.

If the skull has been awash in ocean water for an extended period, the teeth and alveolar bone will appear to have a sandblasted effect. Though teeth were lost postmortem, there may be no indicant sharp ridges.

The dental office is the place of choice for examining, charting, x-raying and photographing the dentition of the skeletonized head. Having the police bring the dry skull to the office conserves the dentist's time and enables him to use regular office equipment, which is more familiar and convenient than portable dental equipment. On completion of the examination, the dental remains are turned over to the medical examiner's office.

The explorer and toothbrush are, usually, all that is necessary for examining the jaws of a completely decomposed head. Prior to examination the teeth can easily be cleaned by rinsing under water or scrubbing with a toothbrush. Especially if the remains were discovered in a dirty area, it may be difficult to examine the teeth unless they have first been thoroughly cleaned.

Since the skull was probably exposed to the elements, amalgam fillings may be tarnished and might be overlooked. Therefore, before charting, the dental examiner should carefully check each tooth with a dental explorer.

The condition of the supporting alveolar bone should be recorded on the chart, since from it can be deduced whether teeth were lost postmortem or antemortem. Moreover, it might be useful as an age determinant, extensive bone loss, generally, indicating age over 40.

When the examination is performed in a hospital, the skull is easily transferred to the x-ray department. The detached skull can be placed in a vertical, horizontal or an oblique position. The dentist taking postmortem x-rays in his own office has the advantage of being able to take them in the regular dental angulations.

Since there is no flesh encasing the jaws, exposure time should be reduced to avoid overexposure of the film (see Chapter 6). If possible, develop x-rays immediately so as to be assured that (1) satisfactory films were obtained, (2) no restorations were overlooked in the examination and (3) all conditions revealed in the x-rays have been noted on the chart.

Case History

Months after a woman was reported missing from her home in central Connecticut, a female skeleton was discovered in a woods near the area where the woman's car had been found shortly after her disappearance. The skull (Fig. 4-4) was brought to the forensic dentist for examination. When the mouth was charted, a comparison with the antemortem dental chart indicated the skeleton was that of the missing woman. Since the antemortem x-rays were bite-wings, postmortem bite-wings were taken. The matching x-rays corroborated the dental charts, and an identification was made (Fig. 4-5).

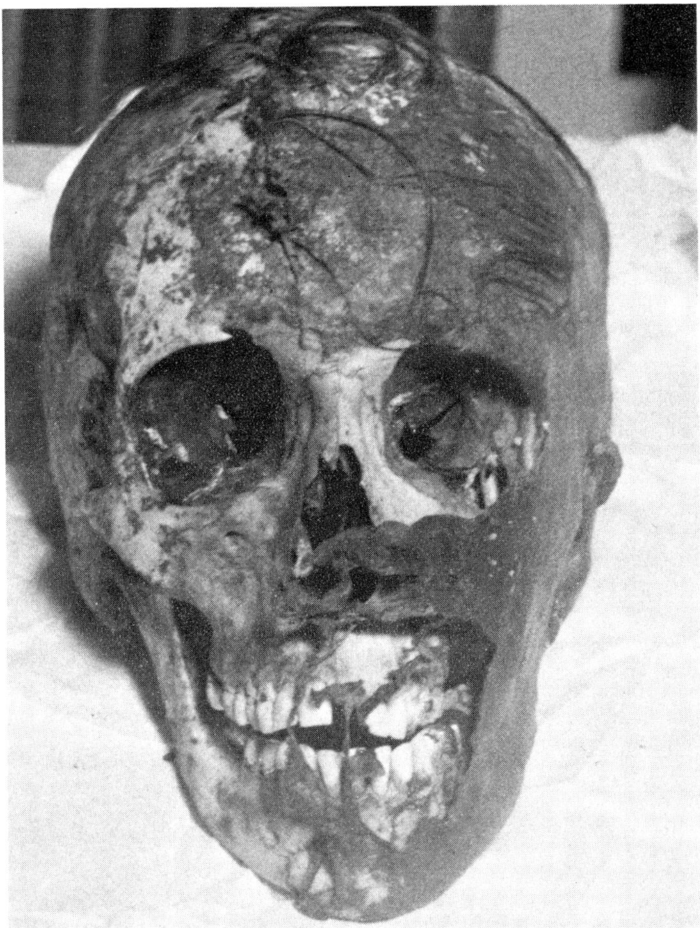

Fig. 4-4. Skull of woman missing from home four months. Mummified skin, covering left side of head, was easily removed by hand, leaving the cranium devoid of soft tissue.

BURNED HEAD

Of all cases of dental identification the burned head is probably the most difficult because of the problems involved in gaining access to the mouth. Attaining access to the mouth may be complicated by the inability to distinguish, especially in the severely burned head, the area of the eyes, nose and lips. There may be no visible mouth; the tissues are hard, crusted and unyielding; and the head may resemble little more than a charred roast of beef.

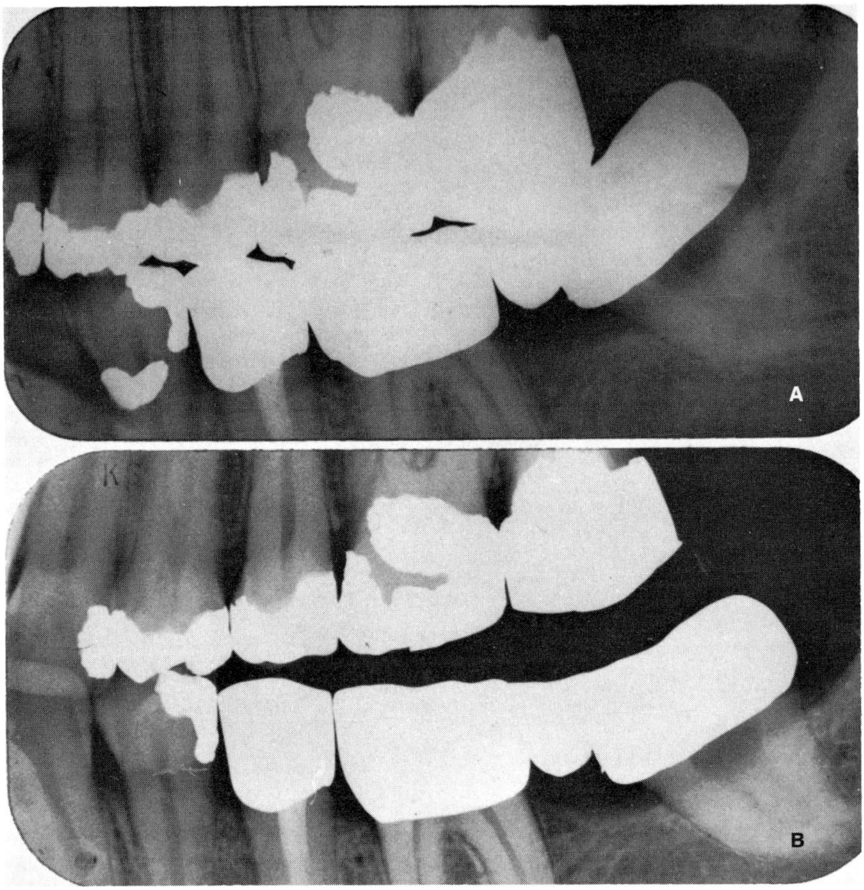

Fig. 4-5. Comparison of antemortem bite-wing x-ray, *A*, and post-mortem bite-wing, *B*, confirmed the identification. Observe the numerous matching details in the two x-rays.

In the severely burned head, it is not unusual for the mouth to be sealed shut. Where the body has been almost completely incinerated, the teeth and mucous membrane, nevertheless, may be unaffected, for the tongue, cheeks and other tissues of the face are excellent insulators, shielding the teeth and periodental tissue from heat and flames.

In the case of the burned head, resection of the jaws is usually indicated for the following reasons:

1. It facilitates examining and charting.

2. The resected jaws are easily taken to a dental office for x-raying in regular dental angulations, simplifying comparison with antemortem x-rays. When the examination is performed in a hospital, there is no problem transferring the jaws to the x-ray department. Hospitals are reluctant, however, to permit moving a dead body intact to the x-ray department.

3. It enables the dentist to take good photographs of the dentition.

4. The dentist can engage in identification procedures away from the odor and atmosphere of the body.

Resecting the Jaws

The sequence of pictures in Figure 4-6, *A* through *O*, demonstrates the techniques for resecting the jaws in a burned head. A body requiring resection of the jaws is, most likely, a closed casket case and not suitable for viewing by relatives or friends (Fig. 4-6*A*). The resection should be done with the permission of the medical examiner.

With a No. 20 blade scalpel, an inverted *V* incision is made on each side of the skull from the commissure of the mouth to the angle of the jaw (Fig. 4-6*B*). If the mouth is obscure, a wide oval incision should be made in the approximate area of the oral cavity. A tissue forceps, large hemostat or the fingers can be used to pull the tissue back to the ascending ramus in order to fully expose the teeth (Fig. 4-6*C*). After removing as much tissue as possible from the mandible (Fig. 4-6*D*), the dentist, rather than disarticulating the temporomandibular joint, here needless and time-consuming, should cut with a Stryker reciprocating bone saw (see Chapter 3) through each side of the mandible (Figs. 4-6*E*, *F* and *G*) at a point distal enough to the most posterior tooth to avoid cutting through tooth structure and damaging the dentition as well as the saw blade. The scalpel is then placed below the angle of the jaw at the inferior border of the mandible and brought upward, cutting away all muscular attachments on each side (Figs. 4-6*H*, *I* and *J*) and freeing the mandible so that it can be lifted out from the skull (Fig. 4-6*K*).

Using a scalpel and tissue forceps, the dentist next removes the facial tissue covering the teeth in the maxilla so that they will be completely visible (Figs. 4-6*L* and *M*). Placing the power bone saw superior to the apical area of the maxillary teeth and cutting through the maxillary bone in an arc from the left side to the right frees the maxilla, enabling it to be disengaged from the skull. This procedure

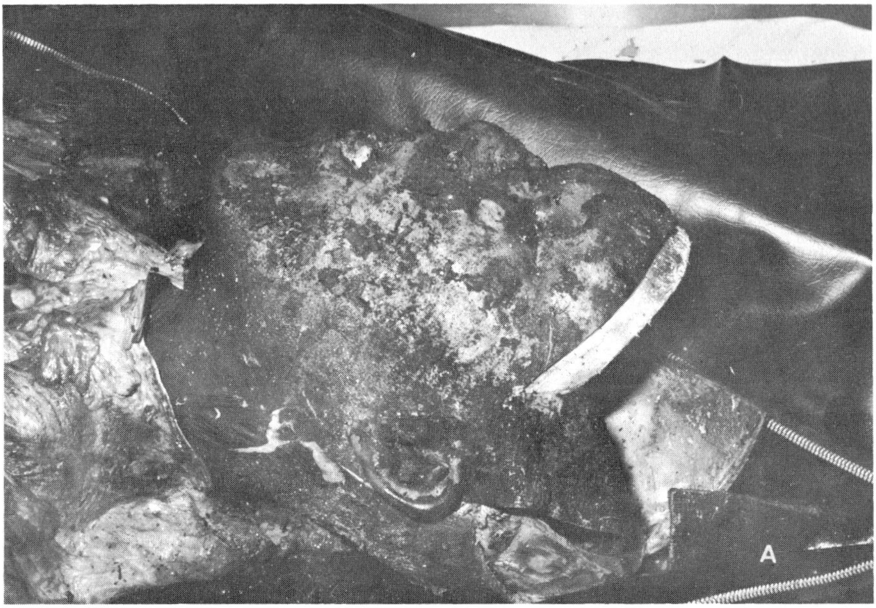

Fig. 4-6. A, Burned head before resection of the jaws. Skull cap was removed previously during autopsy. *B–O,* Resection procedures.

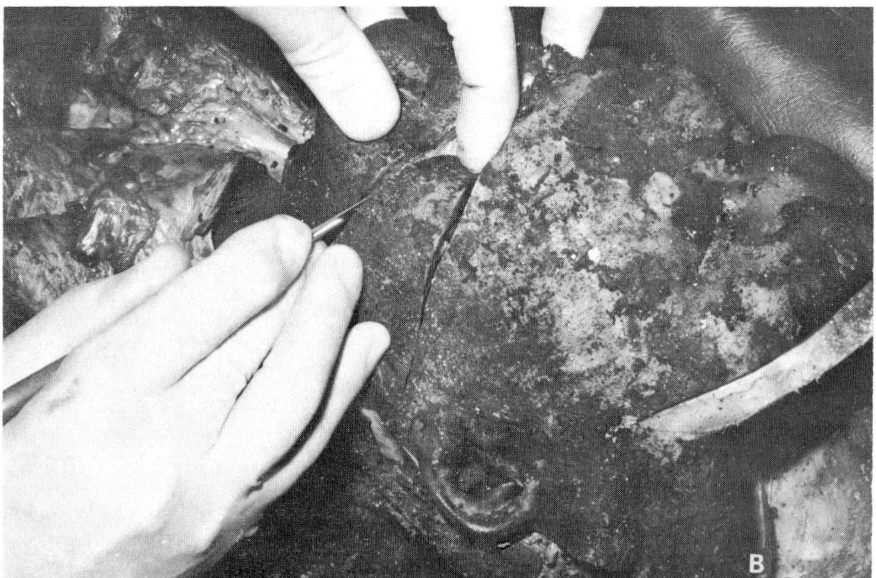

Fig. 4-6B

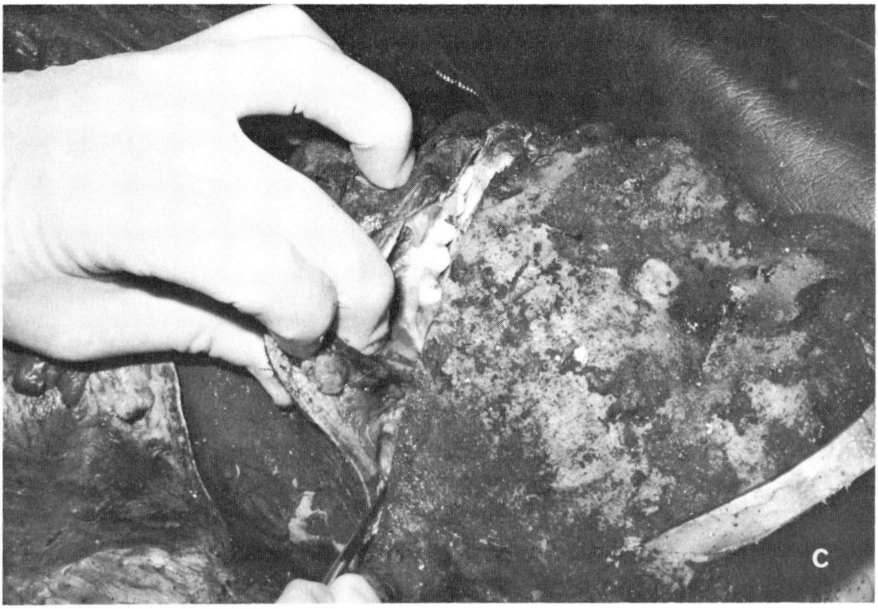

Fig. 4-6C

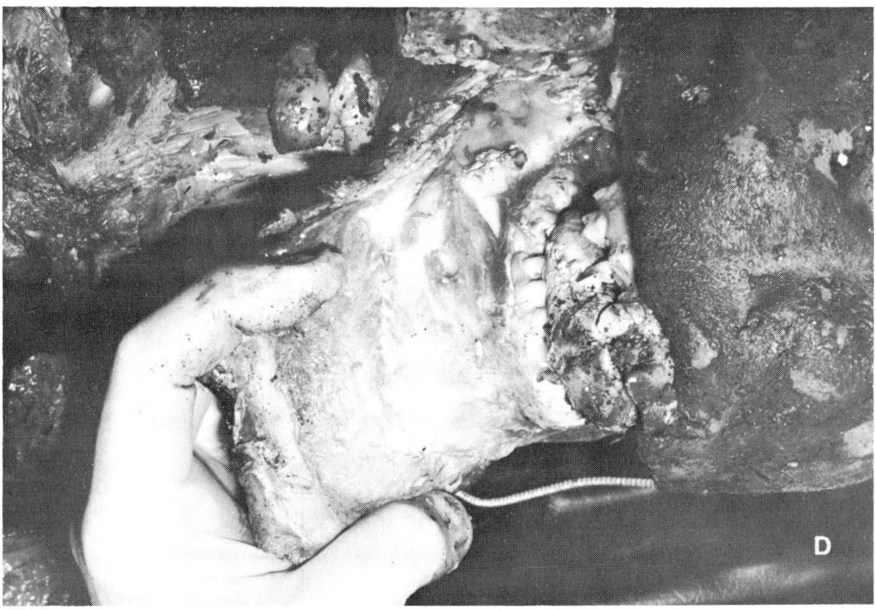

Fig. 4-6D

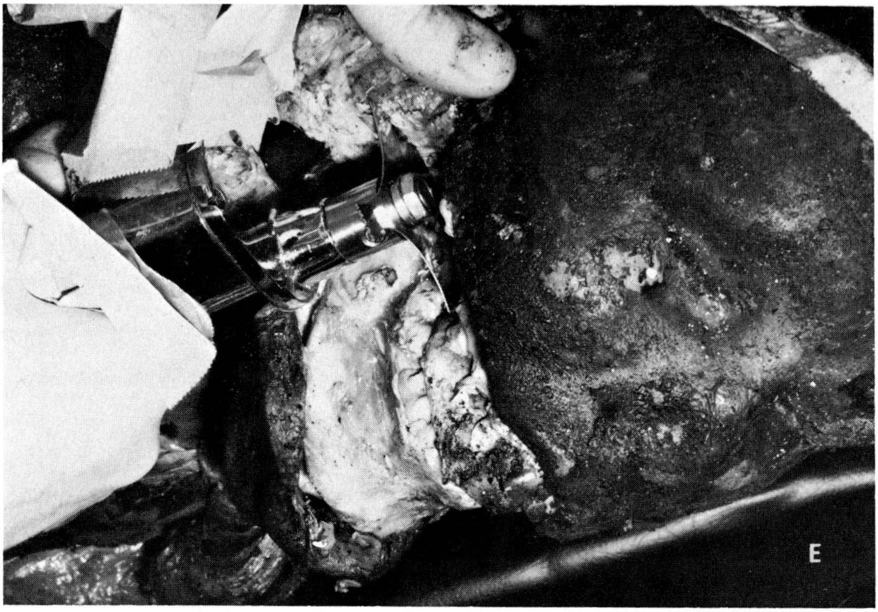

Fig. 4-6E

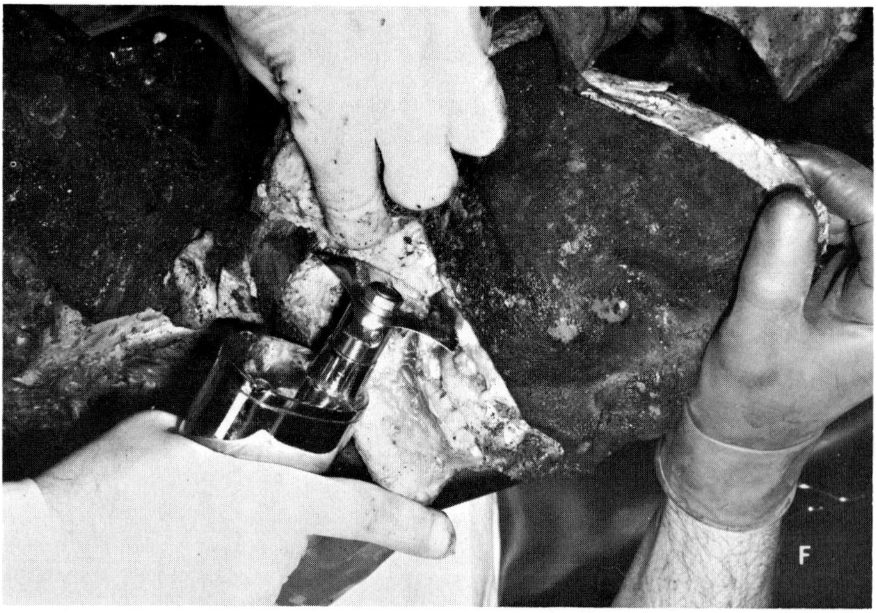

Fig. 4-6F

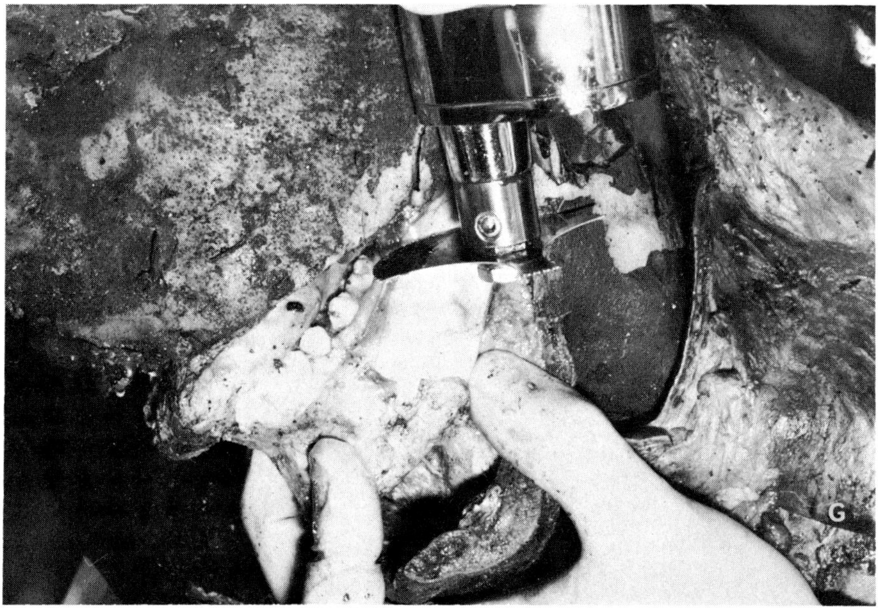

Fig. 4-6G

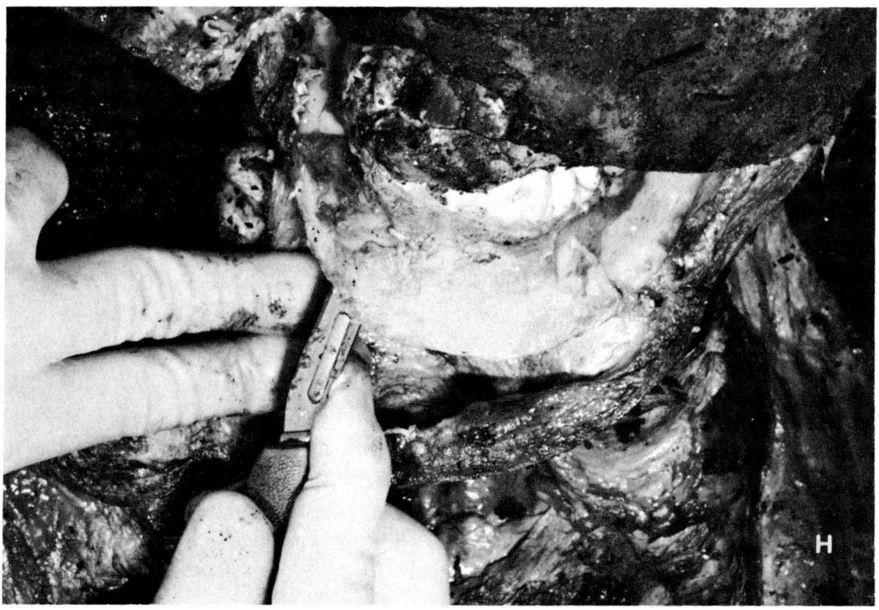

Fig. 4-6H

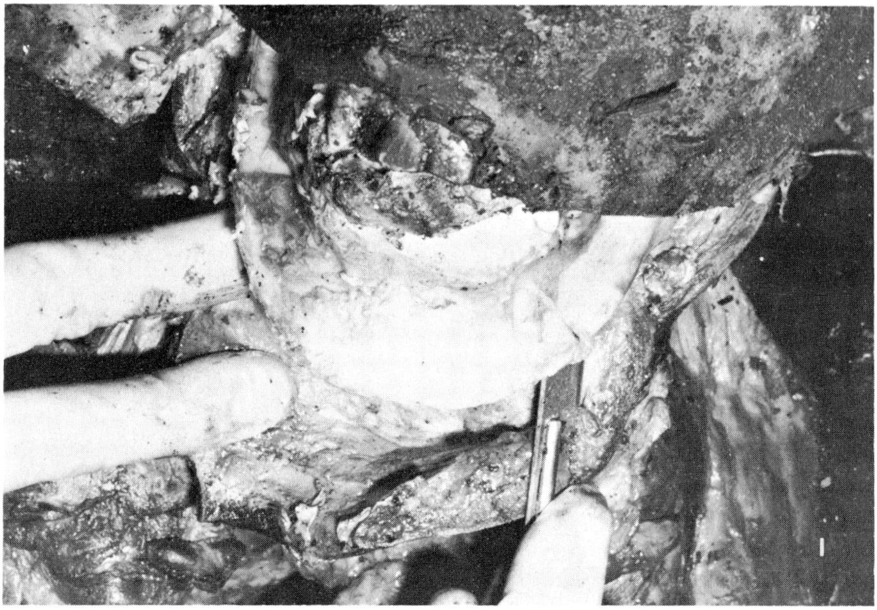

Fig. 4-6I

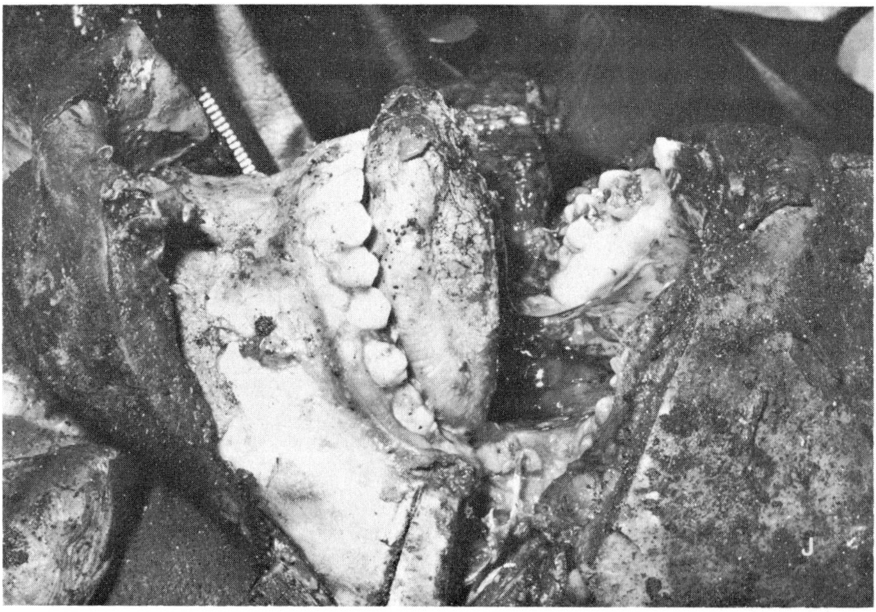

Fig. 4-6J

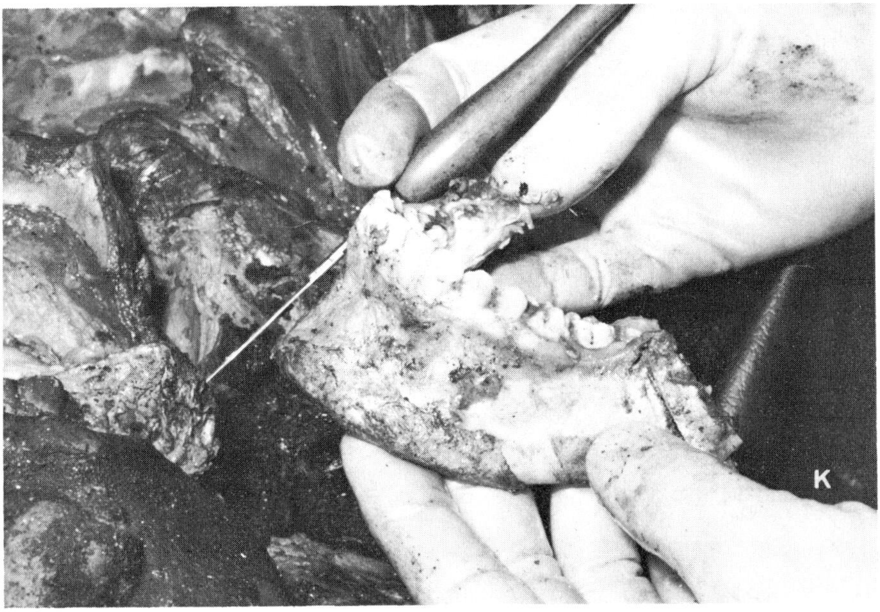

Fig. 4-6K

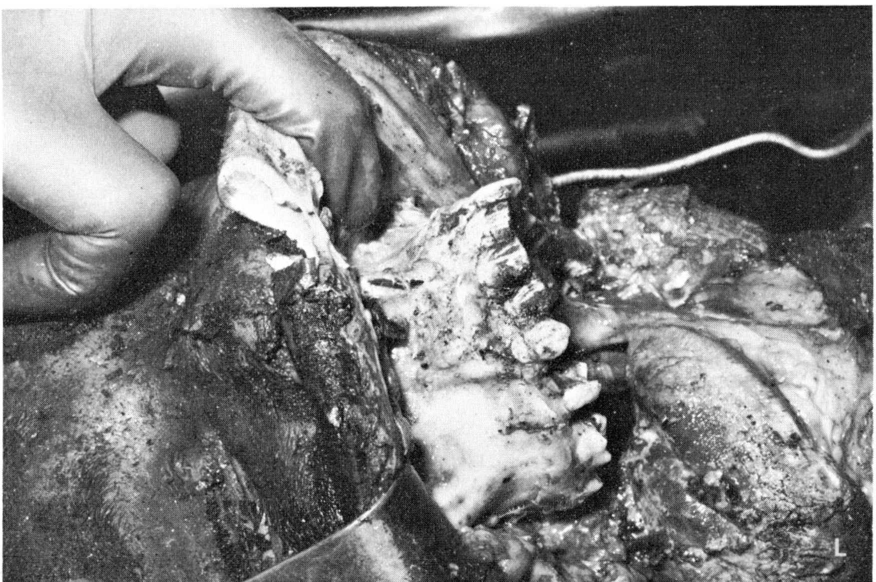

Fig. 4-6L

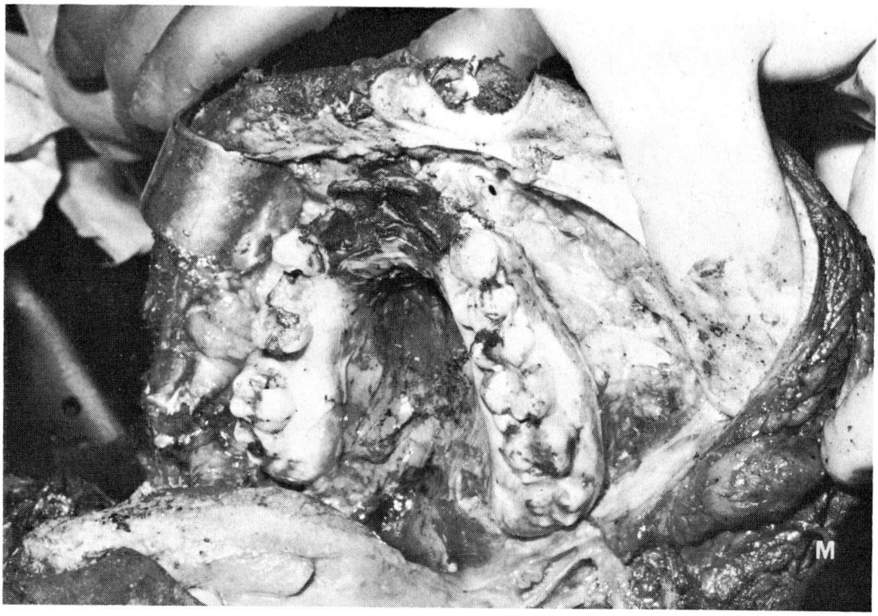

Fig. 4-6M

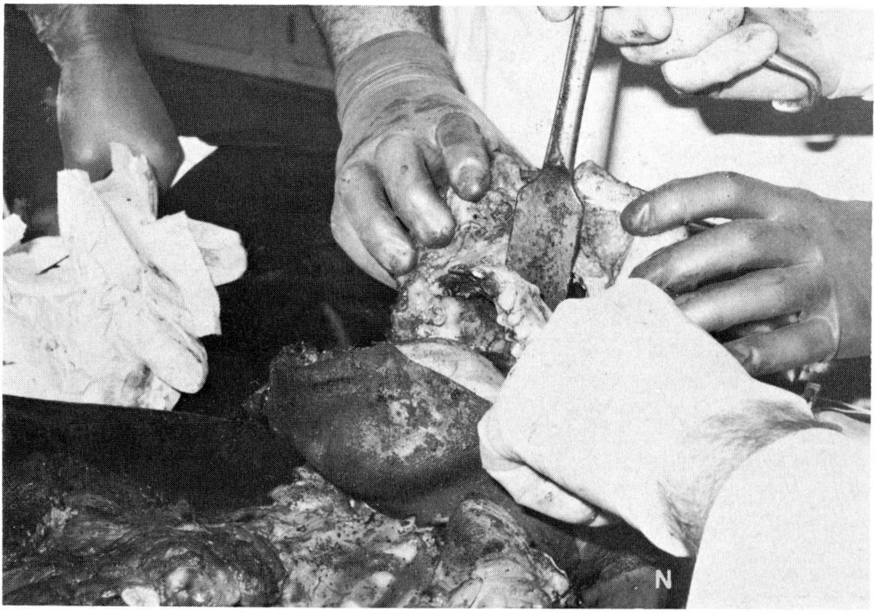

Fig. 4-6N

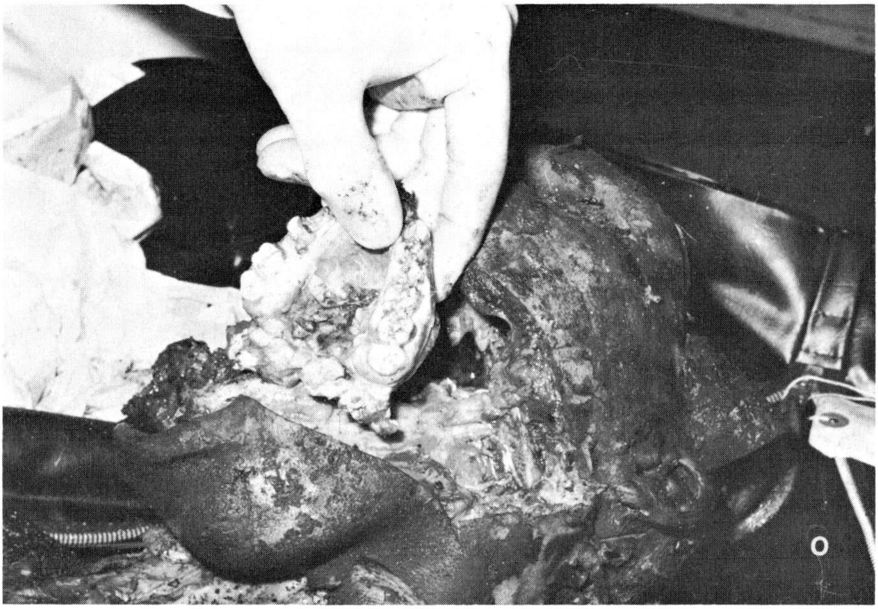

Fig. 4-6O

is not difficult, for the labial plate of bone at the apices of the teeth in the maxilla is thin, and one is actually cutting through the floor of the maxillary sinus. If the saw does not bore completely through a large maxilla, insert the blade of a skull chisel into the saw cut (Fig. 4-6*N*). A sharp blow or two with a hammer, or some other implement, against the chisel handle will sever the maxilla (Fig. 4-6*O*). The detached jaws can now be examined, x-rayed and photographed.

If the resected jaws are to be retained for any length of time, it is advisable that all soft tissue be removed; otherwise, the jaws will have to be kept immersed in formalin or a similar preservative solution. To remove the tissue, soak the jaws for a day or two in a solution of one teaspoon of sodium or potassium hydroxide to one pint of water. (The solution is extremely caustic and must be used with care. Do not let the jaws soak for a prolonged period lest the solution, after consuming the soft tissue, affect bone, teeth and restorations.) When the tissue seems pliable, remove the jaws from the solution and, with a hemostat or tissue forceps, strip the bulk tissue from the bony area. Return the jaws to the solution for another day or so, as required. When the remaining soft tissue has been dissolved, the jaws should be thoroughly washed and air-dried. They can now be retained in a dry state (Fig. 4-7).

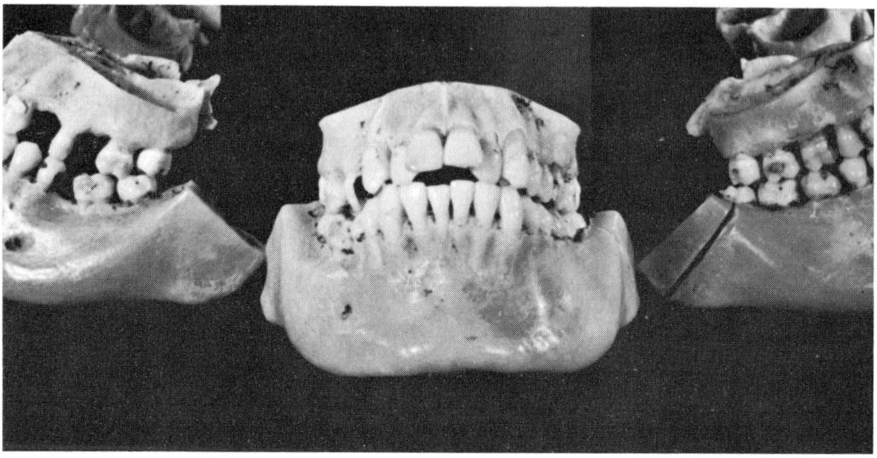

Fig. 4-7. Three-sided view of the resected jaws after all soft tissue has been removed. They can now be retained in a dry state.

Case History

Workers arriving in the morning at a stone quarry in northern Connecticut discovered the remains of a burned out car on the floor of the quarry (Fig. 4-8). A burned human head and hand protruded from the car. The rest of the corpse and all inflammable parts of the car, including the tires, had been incinerated. The victim's remains (Fig. 4-9) were taken to the morgue of a local hospital.

Police speculation was that the car, which was cold, had gone over the cliff early the preceding evening, crashed below and burst into flames. There was a highway twenty-five feet from the cliff, and tire tracks (but no skid marks) were found leading from the road to the edge of the cliff.

From the license plates, the police were able to ascertain the owner of the automobile. Since the owner was missing, it was assumed that it was he who had been consumed in the car.

The only possible means of identification was by the dentition. The family supplied the name of an endodontist (root canal specialist) who had performed root canal therapy on an upper right bicuspid of the missing man. The endodontist was able to furnish x-rays only of that area, showing a molar and bicuspid connected by bridgework.

Since just the right maxillary bicuspid area was of value in the identification, the tissue on the right side of the face in the area of the mouth was removed. With a Stryker reciprocating bone saw,

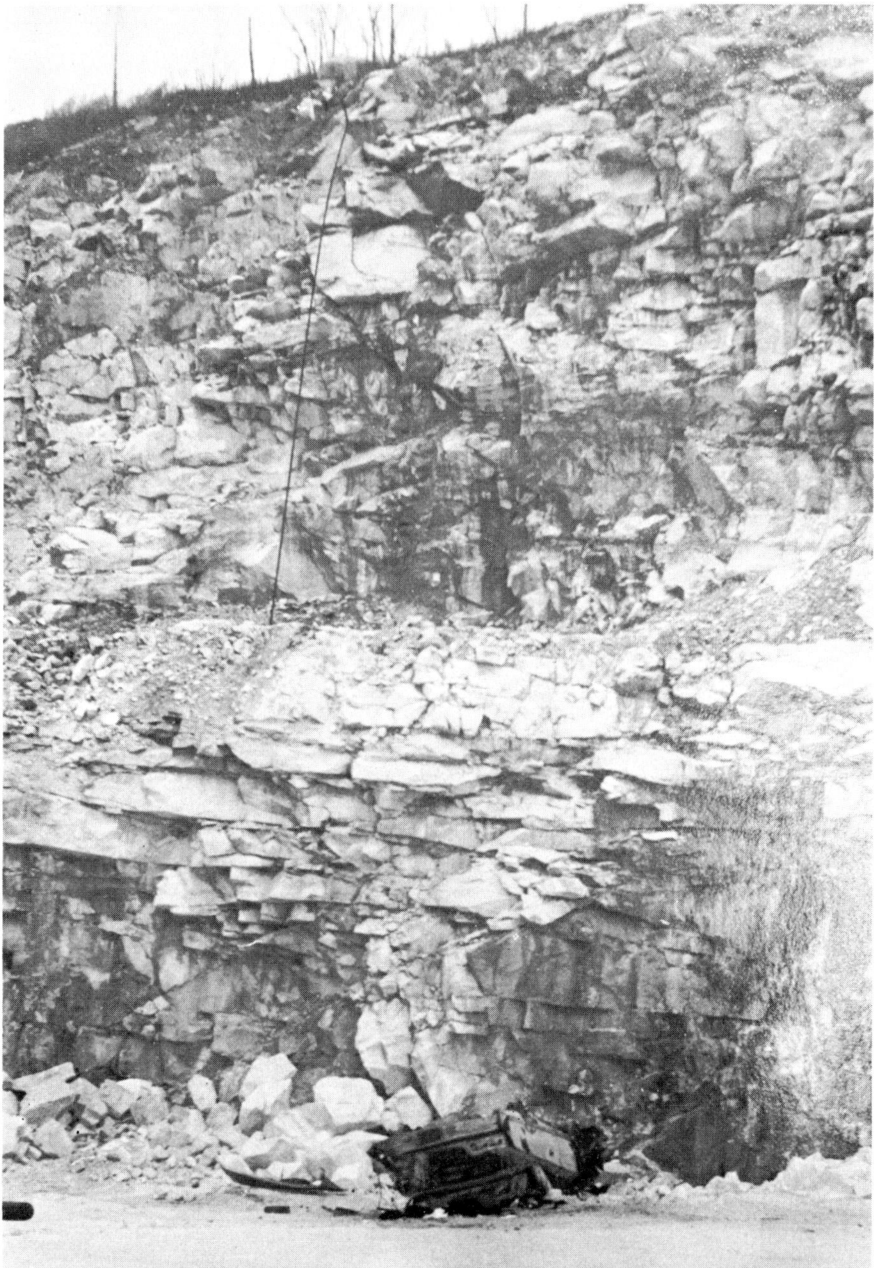

Fig. 4-8. Wreckage of car that went over 108-foot cliff and was found upside down on floor of stone quarry. (Connecticut State Police)

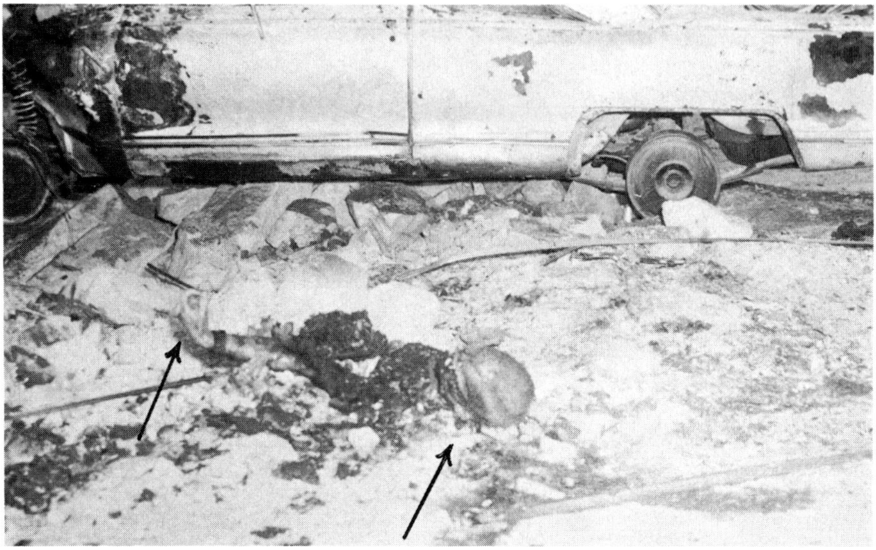

Fig. 4-9. Arrows point to arm and head lying on ground. The rest of the body as well as all inflammable parts of the car, including the tires, had been incinerated. (Connecticut State Police)

the section of maxilla containing the right molar and bicuspid was resected for x-rays (Fig. 4-10). When the postmortem x-ray of the bridgework and dentition matched the antemortem x-ray (Fig. 4-11), identification was made, confirming the assumption that it was the owner who had been incinerated in the car.

During the investigation the police learned that the victim had been a heavy drinker; other than that, the accident was never explained.

MUTILATED HEAD

Mutilation is usually a result of some violent action, such as an airplane crash, a high-speed automobile collision or physical assault. The head may be fragmented, face distorted, and tissues torn—leaving the victim beyond recognition.

Locating the teeth may be a problem, since they may have been dislodged from the jaws. Depending on the cause of fragmentation (e.g., if due to a severe impact type of accident, such as an airplane crash) parts of the body, including the dentition, may be strewn over an area of hundreds of feet, so finely mangled that they may never be retrieved.

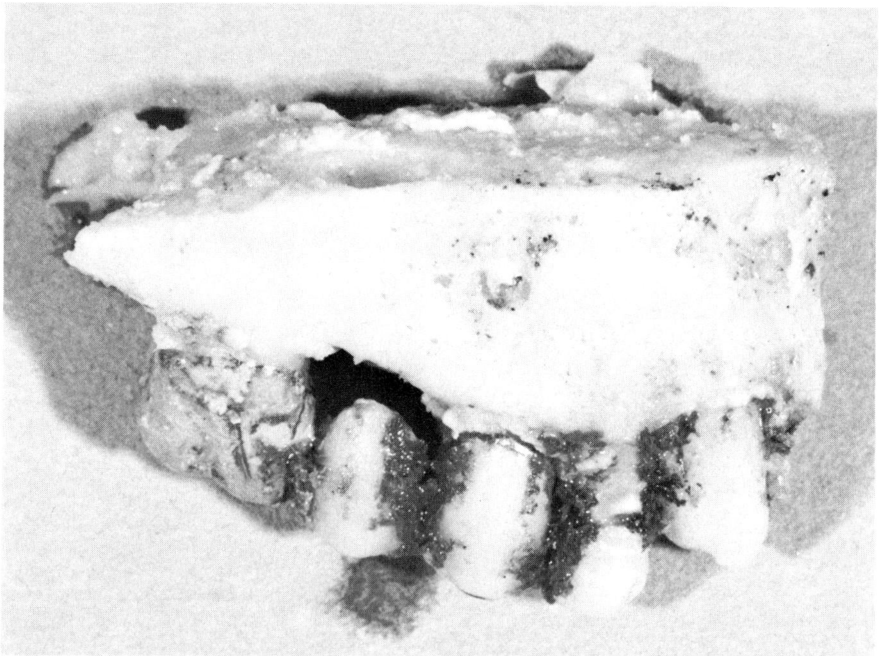

Fig. 4-10. Segment of maxilla resected for postmortem x-rays. Since the only antemortem x-rays available were of the upper right bicuspid area, that section was x-rayed postmortem.

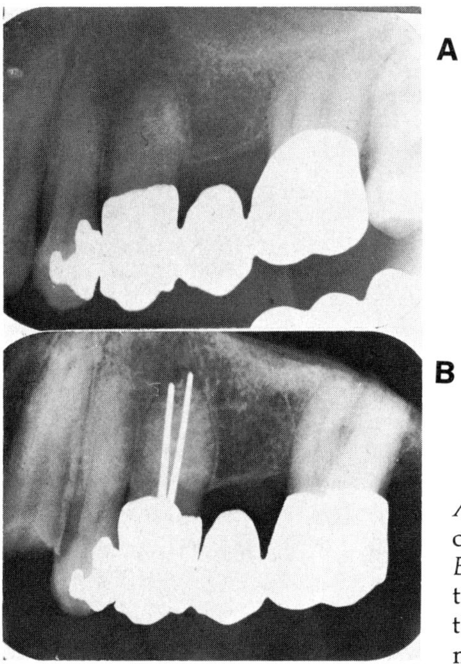

Fig. 4-11. X-rays of bicuspid area. *A*, Antemortem x-ray taken prior to completion of root canal therapy and, *B*, postmortem x-ray of resected section, showing completed root canal therapy. Bridgework and inlay matched in the two pictures.

The first task of the forensic dentist is to locate as many teeth and restorations as possible. This includes making a painstaking search for teeth lying in other organs or entirely separated from the body. In the latter instance, the police can assist by thoroughly searching the recovery area for missing teeth. In the "search-and-find" operation, all particles are scrutinized in an effort to recover, also, pieces of fractured teeth. Since all parts of the jaws and dentition of the mutilated head may not be recovered, care must be exercised in determining whether missing teeth were lost postmortem or antemortem.

In all likelihood the features of the mutilated head are unrecognizable, nor does it lend itself to viewing by relatives or friends, thus eliminating identification by visual means. Because the head is mangled, access to the mouth may not pose a problem as such, for there may well be no definite mouth area. Accordingly, if it is called for, dissection of the fragments with surgical shears, scalpel and hemostats can be blunt, literally cutting and pulling the tissue away from the teeth. If any soft tissue remains on the parts, it will necessitate keeping them in formalin solution or a similar preservative.

All the recovered pieces should be positioned on the examining table in, so far as it is possible, their correct anatomical relationship to each other. Restructuring a semblance to the maxilla and mandible makes it easier to chart, x-ray and photograph.

When the examination is performed in the hospital, the fragments are easily transferred to the x-ray department. If possible, the teeth should be x-rayed in situ. Roots with no crowns remaining should also be x-rayed to record root formation for possible comparison with antemortem x-rays that may be available. If a resection has been done, the same procedures can be carried out in the dental office.

Case History

A nude female body was discovered lying on the side of a limited-access superhighway, about three miles from the nearest entrance. It appeared that the wheels of a truck had passed over the skull, crushing it beyond recognition (Fig. 4-12). The body was removed to a hospital morgue for further examination (Fig. 4-13), which failed to yield any clues to identity, such as rings or scars.

At first, foul play was suspected because of the peculiar location of the body when found. However, a few hours later a man telephoned the police to report that his wife, under treatment for a

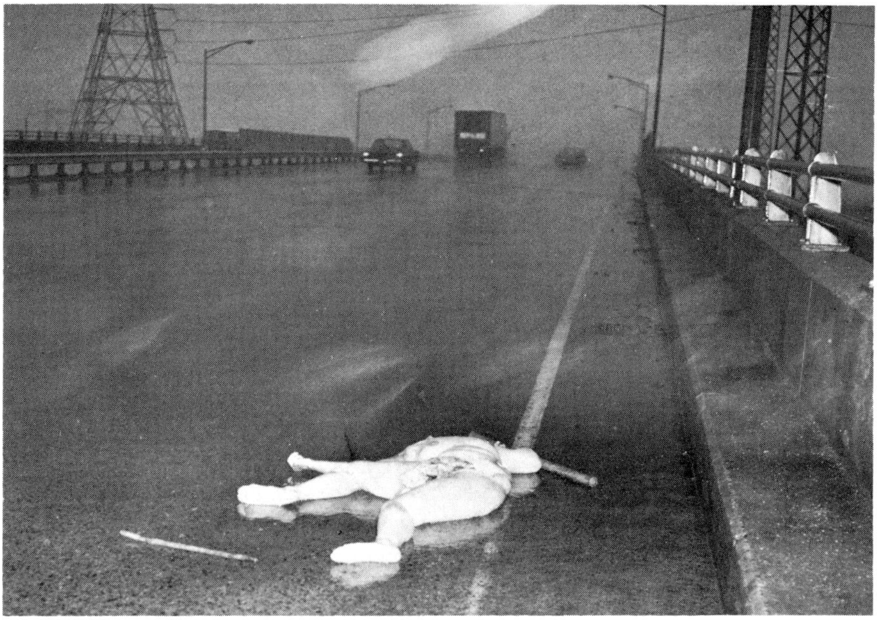

Fig. 4-12. Nude female body found lying at edge of superhighway. Face was crushed beyond recognition. (Connecticut State Police)

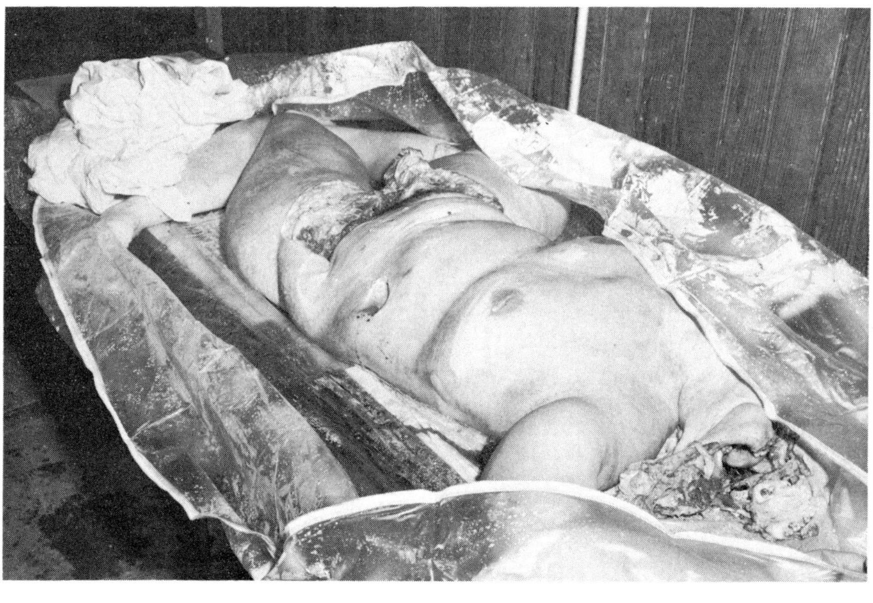

Fig. 4-13. Body in hospital morgue. Observe total mutilation of head. (Connecticut State Police)

mental disorder, was missing. He supplied a description of her and the car in which she had disappeared.

The police located the car on an overpass about three miles from where the body was found. Inside was the woman's clothing.

In order to perform the dental examination, it was necessary to remove the soft tissue from the fractured maxilla and mandible by blunt dissection (Figs. 4-14 and 4-15). Antemortem dental charts and x-rays were furnished. A postmortem x-ray of the lower left molar region matched the antemortem bite-wing x-ray of the same area, enabling an identification to be made (Fig. 4-16).

Police conjecture was that the woman had driven to the overpass intending to throw herself down in front of an oncoming vehicle. Instead, she may have landed just behind the cab area of a trailer truck and, unknown to the driver, was carried about three miles down the highway before rolling off, the rear wheels of the truck passing over her head.

PARTIALLY DECOMPOSED HEAD

The partially decomposed head is probably the most offensive on which to work because of the disagreeable odor. Furthermore, when maggots are present, the sight is repulsive. If the forensic dentist has been forewarned, he can, before entering the autopsy room, stuff No. 2, 1½-inch dental cotton rolls into his nostrils (see Fig. 3-6), apply Noxzema to the lower half of his face and to the protruding ends of the cotton rolls to further shut out any organic odor, and don a surgical mask to retain the cotton rolls in place and prevent the inhalation of bacteria.

The techniques employed for gaining access to the mouth are contingent upon the extent of decomposition present. If the possibility exists of a visual identification, then the head should be treated in the manner described for the head in normal condition—that is, the facial tissue should not be cut. However, if extensive decomposition has taken place and visual identification is not possible, then the orifice of the mouth can be enlarged to make it easier to examine, x-ray and photograph. On each side of the skull, with a No. 20 blade scalpel, cut from the commissure of the mouth straight back through the masseter (cheek) muscle. Generally soft and pliable, the tissue around the dentition can now be easily removed, providing better access to both the maxilla and mandible.

Before the examination, aspiration may be necessary, since the

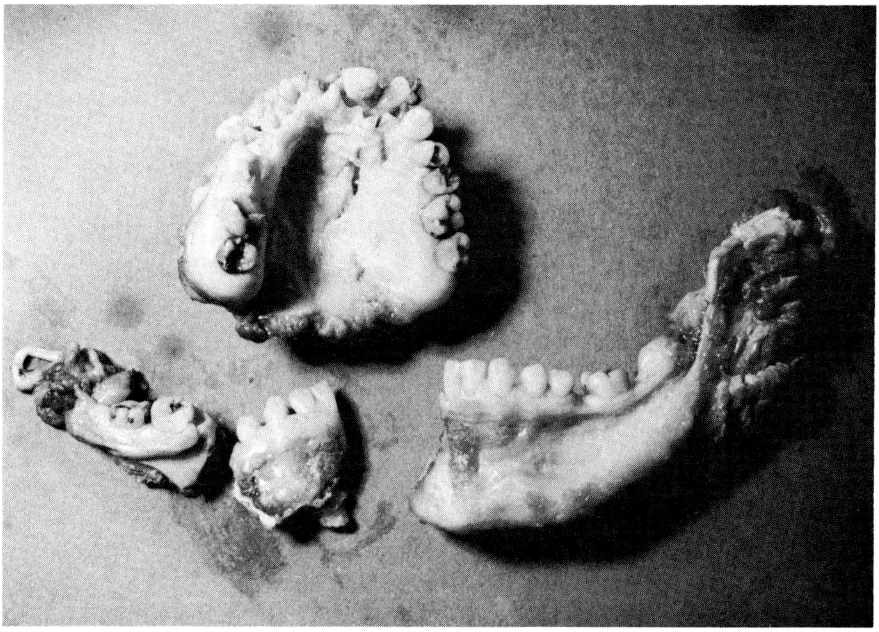

Fig. 4-14. Pieces of the jaws, removed by blunt dissection from mutilated head. Right maxillary teeth (*top*) were sheared at gumline in accident.

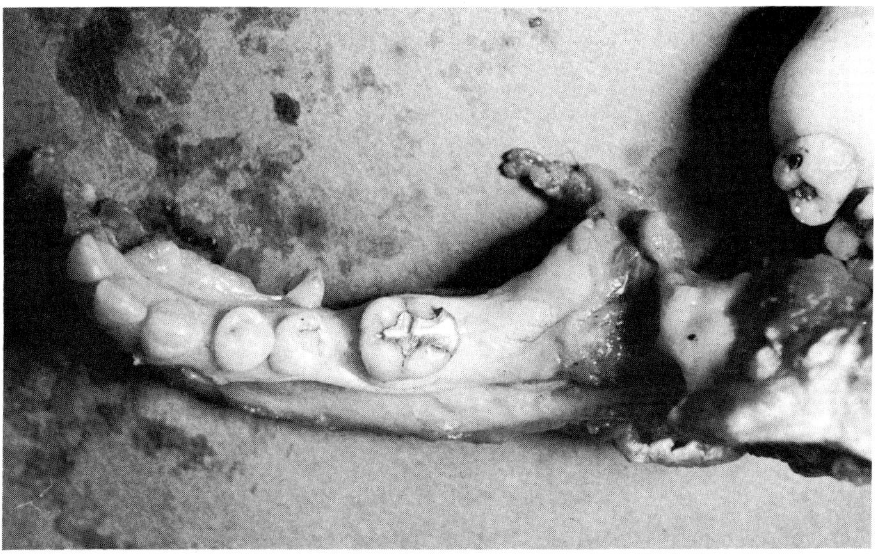

Fig. 4-15. Lower left teeth of victim. Note distal occlusal amalgam in second molar.

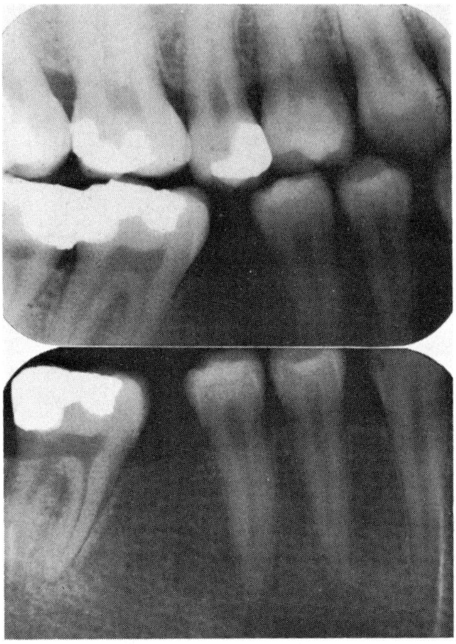

A

B

Fig. 4-16. A, Antemortem and, *B,* postmortem x-rays. Distal occlusal amalgam restoration in lower second molar can be seen in both x-rays.

breakdown of tissue that occurs in the process of physical decomposition can result in fluid accumulation. If there is debris on the teeth, scrub the surfaces with a toothbrush, flush with water, if needed, and wipe clean with a 4 × 4-inch gauze sponge. Clean teeth and a clear field of vision decrease the chance of errors in examining and charting.

If good access has been created by surgical intervention, the examination can now be performed with the aid of a dental explorer and mirror. Almagam fillings are more apparent in the partially decomposed head than in the skeletonized, since they have not yet tarnished.

If complete antemortem records, including x-rays, are available at the time of the examination, it may be possible to make an identification without postmortem x-rays. Because of accompanying odors and the possibility of contamination, it is probably not feasible to move the partially decomposed head from the autopsy room. Therefore, if x-rays are needed and no portable x-ray machine is available, it will be necessary to resect the jaws, removing loose tissue, and, discreetly, transfer them to the hospital x-ray department. The resection procedure is similar to that for the burned head, though less laborious in those instances where the decomposed tissue is soft and pliant. If the body is to be buried without identity having been established, it may be deemed desirable to resect and retain the jaws on the possibility that they could be useful for identification at a later time.

Case History

At 1:45 A.M., in a driving rainstorm, a pilot and friend took off from Long Island in a private plane, heading toward the Connecticut shoreline. Before departing, they had been drinking heavily at the airport bar, according to a third drinking companion, who had chosen not to accompany them for the ill-fated flight. The plane and both occupants disappeared.

About six months later, the remains of an aircraft were recovered in the nets of a lobster fisherman. Divers dispatched to the area located the missing plane and one body. Underwater, they placed the body in a waterproof sack, which was brought to the surface and put into another waterproof sack for transfer to a mortuary. The body was thought to be that of the lost pilot.

Pumping out the contents of the inner sack discharged an assortment of marine life that had been swimming around in the abdominal cavity. The head was both decomposed and mutilated, leading to the conjecture that the victim had probably struck the windshield when the plane crashed into the ocean.

Extensive decomposition and mutilation made it impossible to recognize landmarks (eyes, nose, mouth, ears) and necessitated groping for pieces of shattered jawbone and teeth (Fig. 4-17). The soft tissue then had to be cut away from the hard structures in order to expose the dentition. After two hours of tedious labor only a few of the anterior teeth were found. The forensic dentist, taking into account that following an airplane crash it is possible for teeth and other structures of the anatomy to be far removed from the body proper, concluded that all of the teeth in the sack had probably been recovered (Fig. 4-18).

The pilot's widow telephoned his dentist, who had no x-rays and could furnish only a sketchy description of the dentistry he had performed, explaining that the actual dental records, written in a "personal code," would be unintelligible. Most of the operative work had been done on anterior teeth that were not recovered with the body. Furthermore, the recovery of both maxillary third molars refuted his claim that he had extracted an upper third molar (Fig.

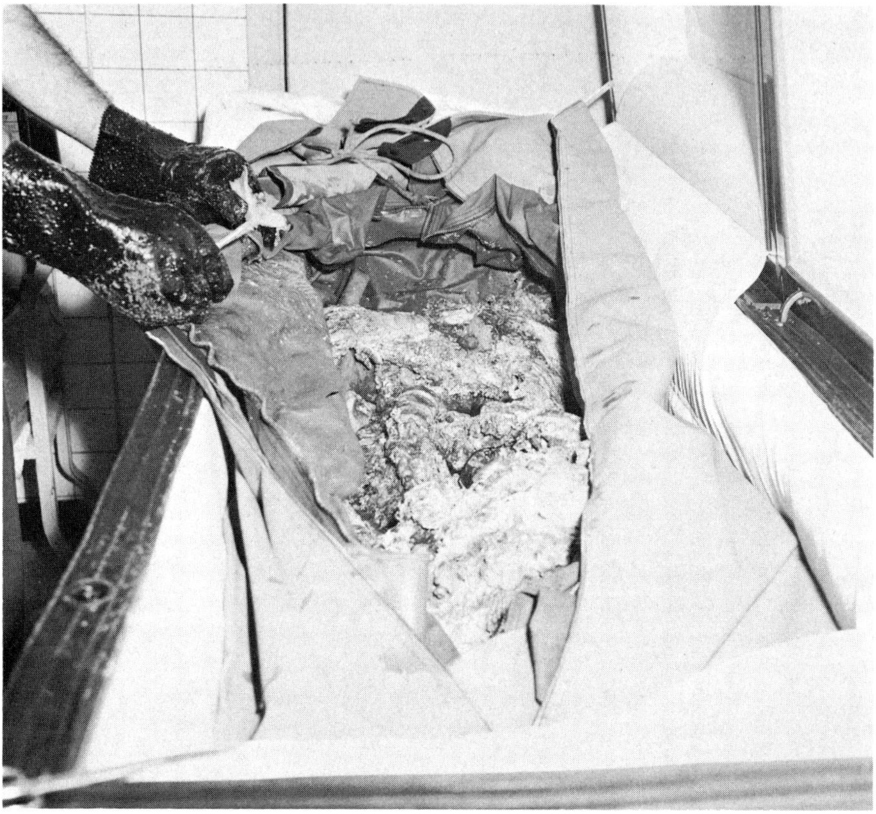

Fig. 4-17. Remains of victim who died in airplane crash in Long Island Sound. Body was both decomposed and mutilated. Dentist probing in casket for pieces of jawbone and teeth is wearing heavy body-recovery gloves for protection against penetration by sharp fragments. (Connecticut State Police)

4-19). The inadequacy and inaccuracy of the antemortem information made it valueless for use in identification.

Then the thought arose that perhaps the body was that of the passenger in the plane. However, dental records disclosed that he had worn full upper and lower dentures.

Failing to find a record of military service, the investigating officer, on checking criminal files, discovered that the pilot, ten years before, had been sentenced to State Prison for one to three years. The prison dental record, made at the time of his entry, showed some teeth marked as both missing and filled. Such discrepancies precluded its use for identification.

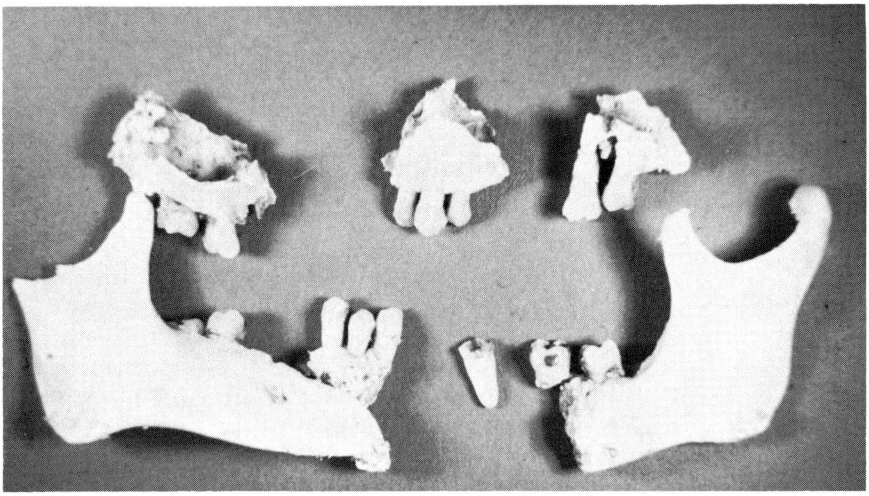

Fig. 4-18. After a two-hour search these were the only teeth recovered from the sack in the casket.

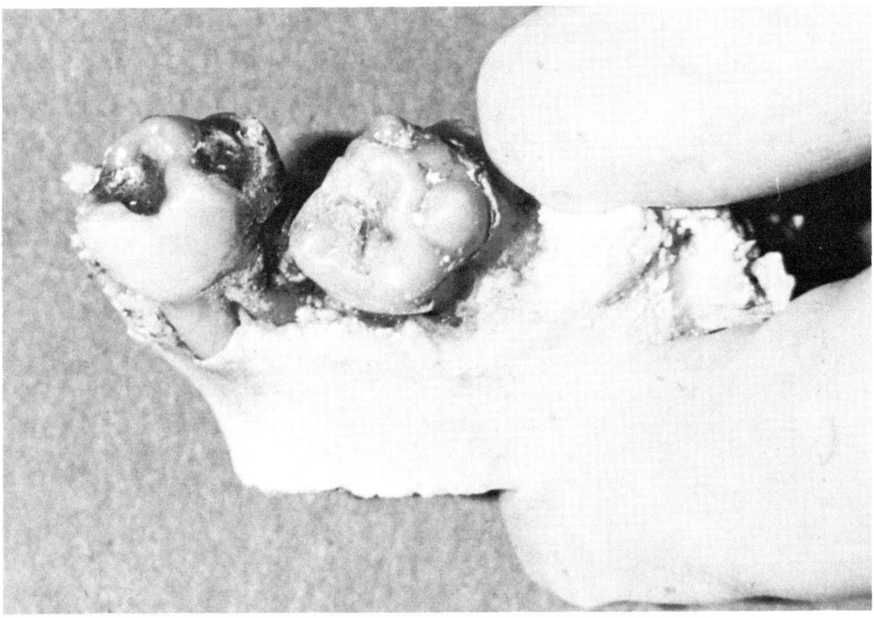

Fig. 4-19. Upper first and third molars recovered from the casket. Although pilot's dentist claimed he had extracted an upper third molar, both maxillary third molars were recovered.

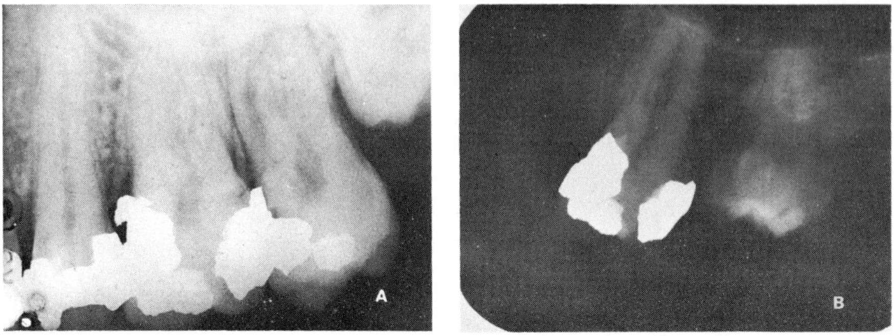

Fig. 4-20. A, The only antemortem x-ray available of missing pilot, taken ten years before his disappearance. Note the three restorations in the first molar, on the mesial, occlusal and distal surfaces. Although faded and poorly preserved, the image was adequate for comparison purposes. *B,* Postmortem x-ray of pilot. The third molar had drifted down into the space left by extraction of the second molar. The three restorations in the first molar matched the three restorations seen in the antemortem x-ray.

However, unearthed in prison files was a single periapical x-ray of the upper molar area, showing the first, second and third molars (Fig. 4-20*A*). Since that area of the mouth had been recovered from the body, a postmortem x-ray (Fig. 4-20*B*) was taken for comparison with the prison x-ray. The x-rays showed the same three fillings in the upper first molar. Furthermore, the postmortem x-ray revealed that the pilot's personal dentist had extracted, in actuality, an upper second molar, not a third molar. The third molar, probably impacted at the time, later drifted down into the space left by the extraction of the second molar. Thus a single antemortem x-ray and considerable sleuthing contributed to the identification of the pilot's body.

5 Postmortem Records

After access has been gained to the mouth, the examination and charting are begun. The essential difference between the postmortem examination and the routine dental examination performed in the office of the general practitioner is that the latter is concerned, primarily, with pathological conditions, such as caries and other oral diseases, whereas the postmortem examination is, basically, a search for identifying characteristics in the oral cavity. The information garnered from a dental examination of the deceased is contained in the postmortem dental record.

Various methods are used to record the postmortem dental data. The kinds of postmortem dental records normally made use of are (1) the diagrammatic chart, (2) verbal charting, (3) tape recording, (4) x-rays, (5) photographs and (6) models. Although they corroborate and reinforce each other, it is unlikely that all the kinds of postmortem dental records will be utilized in a case. Moreover, under certain circumstances some would be preferable to others.

Since the results of the postmortem examination will be compared with antemortem records, the method used to record the postmortem dental data may be predicated on the form, content, and extent of the antemortem information that has been obtained prior to the postmortem examination (i.e., if the only antemortem record is an x-ray showing three teeth, then a postmortem x-ray should be taken of the same teeth—possibly eliminating the need for other postmortem procedures). Where antemortem records have not yet been secured, the postmortem record should be as complete as possible, since there is no way of knowing which will be the contributory factors to a dental identification. Injury to the dentition due to mutilation or charring may preclude comprehensive postmortem recording.

Case History

A pilot flying alone in a single-engine Cessna 185 from Godfrey Field, Leesburg, Virginia, to Bradley International Airport crashed in evening rain and fog into the side of Talcott Mountain in Simsbury, Connecticut (Fig. 5-1). The dead pilot was mutilated and burned beyond recognition. On the tail of the plane, the only section left intact, were the identification numbers.

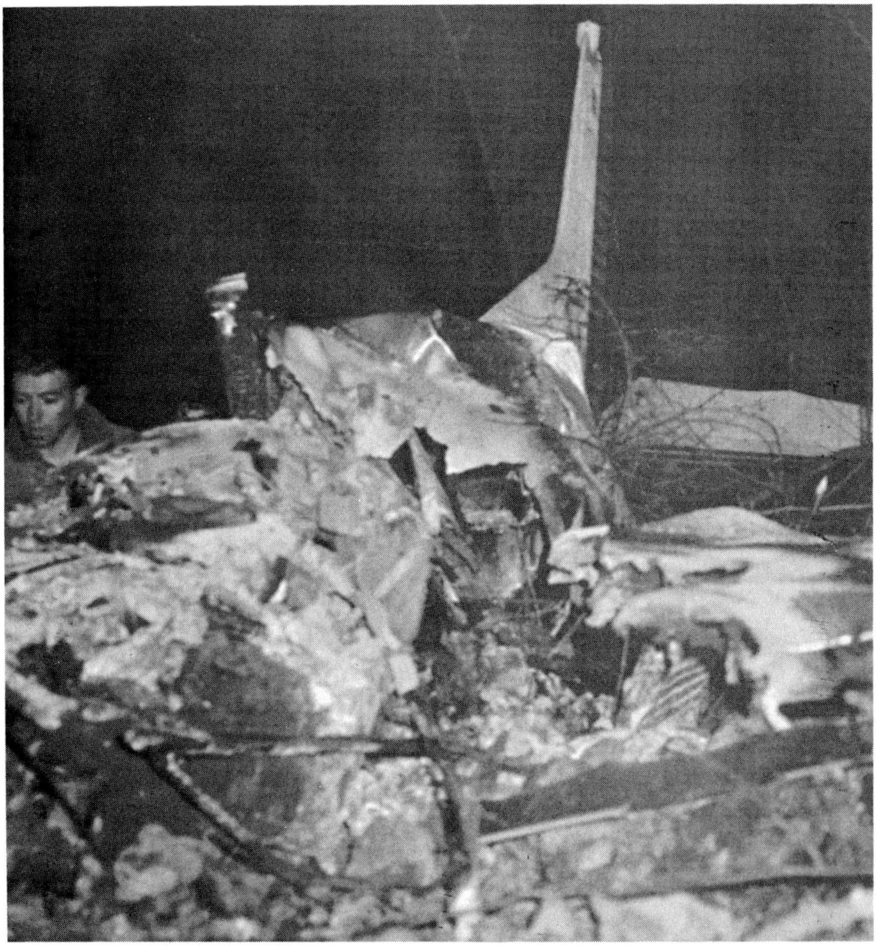

Fig. 5-1. Only the tail section remained of a light plane that crashed into Talcott Mountain in Connecticut, killing the pilot. (Simsbury Police Department)

The next day, the pilot's brother-in-law furnished the name of the victim's dentist in Leesburg, whose only record of the pilot was a single periapical x-ray of the lower right posterior teeth. After reading the x-ray over the telephone to the forensic odontologist, the dentist agreed to send it by airmail to Hartford for verification.

All of the victim's teeth were fractured except for the lower right quadrant. Since it was the only part of the dentition that had been x-rayed antemortem, according to the Leesburg dentist, that segment of teeth was resected by the odontologist and taken to a local dental office for x-rays (Figs. 5-2 and 5-3).

Meanwhile, the odontologist was notified by telephone from Virginia that friends of the deceased were driving to Washington, D.C., to make contact with an Allegheny Airlines flight to Bradley International Airport. At a cost of $21, an envelope containing the single x-ray was ticketed aboard in Allegheny's parcel delivery service. A Simsbury policeman met the plane at Bradley and transported the envelope to the funeral home where the odontologist was waiting. Only three hours after the film left Virginia, a positive identification

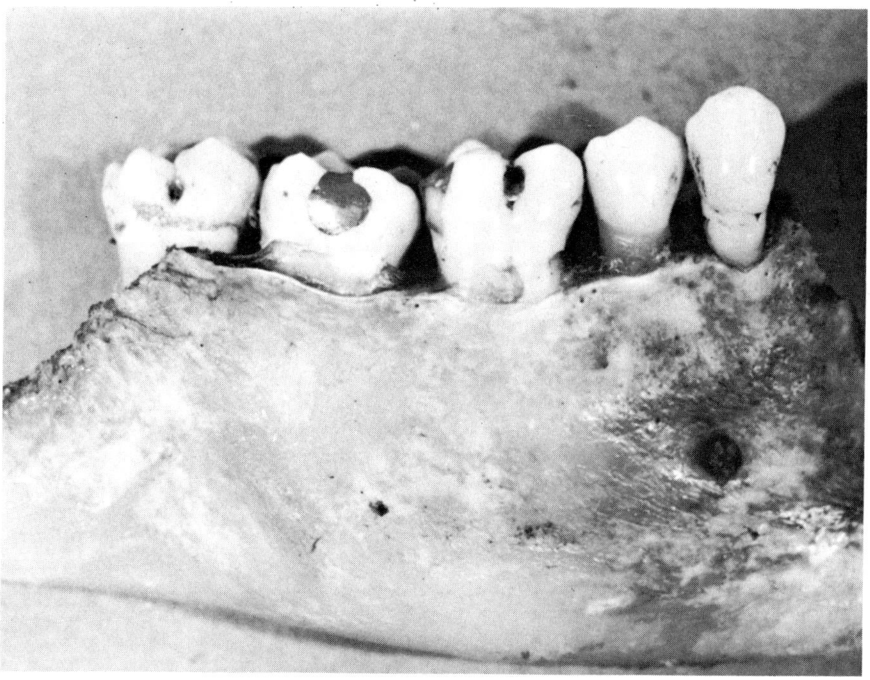

Fig. 5-2. Fragment of mandible resected for x-raying.

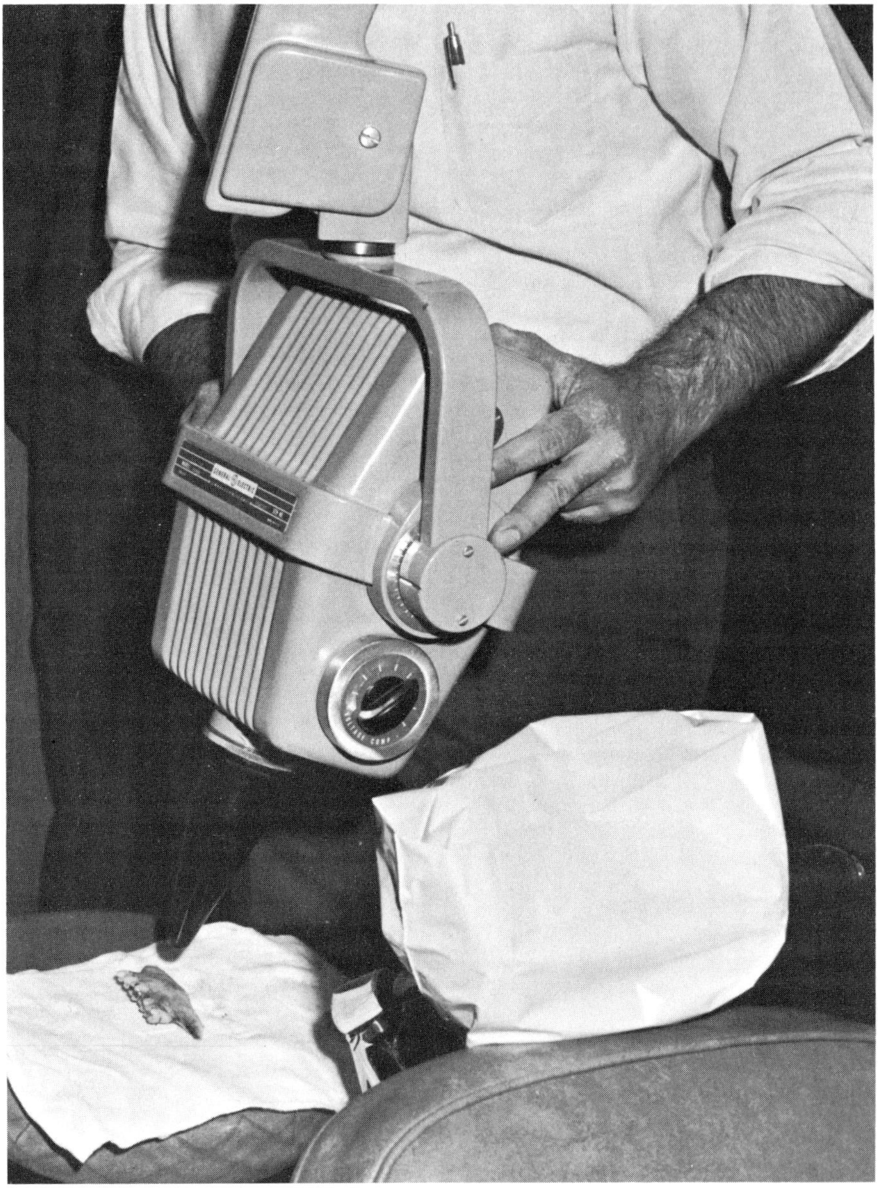

Fig. 5-3. Mandibular fragment being x-rayed in local dental office. Although the jaw fragment has been placed horizontally, the position of the film and teeth and the angulation of the x-ray cone are in the same relationship to each other as would be expected in the antemortem x-ray. Since the section was devoid of soft tissue, exposure time was decreased by half. (Simsbury Police Department)

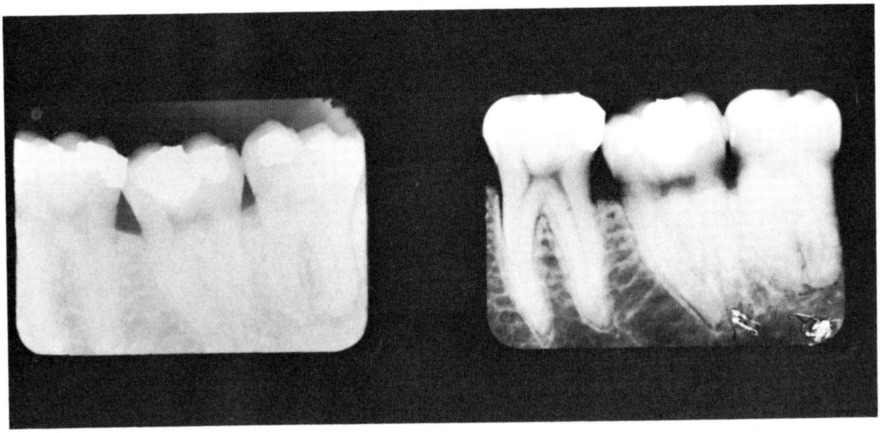

Fig. 5-4. Antemortem (*left*) and postmortem x-rays. Observe similarities in crown and root formations and in restorations, seen in the two x-rays.

was able to be made on the basis of a single antemortem x-ray compared with a matching postmortem x-ray (Fig. 5-4).

METHODS FOR RECORDING POSTMORTEM INFORMATION

The Diagrammatic Chart

The pictorial representation of the dentition is the most commonly used type of dental record. Of the many variations of diagrammatic dental charts available, the one preferred for use in dental identification has the thirty-two teeth of the human mouth pictured anatomically, providing views of the tooth surfaces (see Figs. 5-5 and 5-9). Comprehensive dental notations based on a survey of the oral cavity are made on the chart (Fig. 5-5*B*). The advantage of the anatomical drawing over other sorts of diagrammatic charts (see Fig. 8-2) is that it permits the dentist to sketch in a truer delineation of the shapes and sizes of restorations. The prevalence of many different systems for charting the human mouth is an unfortunate complication.

As a general rule, the condition of the mouth at the time of the postmortem examination is recorded on the chart and in x-rays and photographs unless, as was mentioned earlier, the antemortem records clearly eliminate the need for the total procedure. The diagrammatic chart affords a compact, representative view of the state of the entire dentition, thus facilitating comparison with antemortem records—of particular significance in a mass disaster, which involves multiple victims and, in all probability, different kinds of antemortem records.

Verbal Charting

Basically a detailed, written word-description of the dental examination, verbal charting is more time-consuming to execute than diagrammatic charting and less easily compared with antemortem records. Although often unwieldy, the verbal description has two seeming advantages over the diagrammatic chart: (1) At the present time, it is more readily transmitted; (2) In the diagrammatic chart there is more chance of error from mismarking than in verbal charting where the teeth are designated by their specific names.

Tape Recording

Oral charting by means of a portable cassette tape recorder, with a foot switch for hands-free operation, if necessary, can be done simultaneously with the postmortem examination. An immediate replay of the tape enables the dentist to review his procedure while checking it directly against the dentition. Moreover, because a tape can be played back repeatedly at will, it can be used at any time to verify written records, such as diagrammatic and verbal charting.

X-rays

Because they accurately reveal anatomical landmarks and the greatest number of other details (bone support, root formation, interior configuration of restorations, etc.), x-rays are probably the most exact and reliable record of the mouth. Consequently, under certain circumstances, a dental identification can be made solely on the basis of a single antemortem x-ray compared with a corresponding postmortem x-ray, as shown in the preceding case history.

It is helpful to have antemortem x-rays on hand at the time of the postmortem examination, inasmuch as they would determine the kind of x-rays to be taken of the deceased. A careful effort should be made by the dentist, x-ray technician or trained assistant—whoever is taking the postmortem dental x-rays—to match as closely as possible the view of the dentition seen in the antemortem x-rays.

Since bite-wings are the most commonly used x-rays in routine dentistry, they are frequently used postmortem for comparative purposes in dental identification. In a single exposure of each side of the mouth, bite-wings afford a view, showing caries and restorations, of most of the posterior teeth. If the antemortem x-rays are periapicals, then matching periapical views should be taken postmortem. Although occlusal film does not reveal all the details that can be seen in the bite-wing and periapical, it is useful, nonetheless, where there is restricted access to the mouth, since it usually can be inserted despite the oral stricture. At the present time it is, generally, not feasible to use standard panoramic equipment for postmortem roentgenograms. All the details revealed in the postmortem x-rays should also be noted on the postmortem dental chart.

Photographs

Postmortem photographs of the head, face and oral region should include an occlusal view of the maxilla and the mandible and an anterior view of the dentition with, if possible, the jaws in occlusion. Photographs reinforce the charting (see Chapter 7).

Models

Rarely are postmortem models utilized as evidence for dental identification, although it is possible that the circumstances of a case might warrant taking impressions in alginate of the mouth of the deceased, particularly where the antemortem records consist of study or prosthetic models.

CONDITIONS TO BE NOTED IN POSTMORTEM CHARTING

The postmortem examination and charting must be meticulously done, since in all probability, there is only one contact with the body. The state of the oral cavity in general and of the dentition and its supporting structure in particular should be duly noted, and the following details recorded on the postmortem Dental Identification Record form (Fig. 5-5*A*).

Missing Teeth

A simple way to indicate teeth missing from the victim is to mark the corresponding teeth on the diagrammatic chart with an *X*. It is

DENTAL IDENTIFICATION RECORD

Outline all caries and restorations on chart.
Shade in restorations only. See code below.

Police Case No.____________________
M. E. Case No.____________________
City__________________Date________

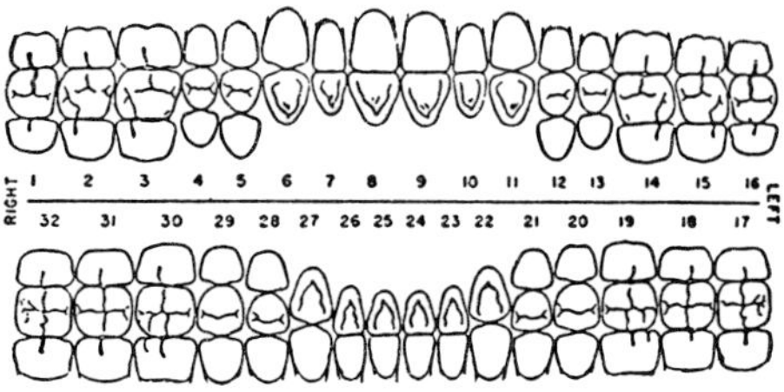

Circumstances requiring examination:

Site of examination:

Jaw Relationship
- ☐ Normal
- ☐ Protruding upper jaw
- ☐ Protruding lower jaw

A	Amalgam filling
G	Gold filling
S	Silicate or plastic filling
X	Tooth missing
LPM	Lost postmortem
PC	Porcelain crown
GC	Gold crown
SC	Steel crown
VC	Veneer crown
B	Fixed bridge (use brackets beginning and ending with supporting teeth)
PD	Partial denture
FD	Full denture

Prosthetic Appliances
- Maxilla
  - ☐ Fixed Bridge
  - ☐ Partial Denture
  - ☐ Full Denture
- Mandible
  - ☐ Fixed Bridge
  - ☐ Partial Denture
  - ☐ Full Denture

Describe prosthetic appliances:

This box to be filled in if identification is made. Date________ Time______
Name of Deceased________________
Street and No.________________
City__________ State______
Birthdate__________ Age______
Sex__________ Race______

Abnormalities and other oral conditions:

Postmortem dental photographs Yes ☐ No ☐
Postmortem dental x-rays Yes ☐ No ☐

Name and Address of Examiner:

Antemortem records obtained from
Name________________
Street and No.________________
City________________
State________________
Area Code________Tel.________
Describe antemortem records:

Signature of Examiner

Name of Investigating Officer

Additional notes on back Yes ☐ No ☐

SP-144-C Rev. 1972

A

Fig. 5-5. Dental Identification Record used by the Connecticut State Police. This basic form has been employed successfully in over 365 postmortem dental examinations, including a mass disaster. Concise but comprehensive, and without cumbersome instructions, the one-page form is easily executed and readily compared with other matter. In addition, it can be quickly reproduced on a copying machine and transmitted on the Xerox Telecopier, advantages that are particularly important in a mass disaster. *A,* At the onset of a case, since there is no name for the victim, the only designation may be the Police Case

DENTAL IDENTIFICATION RECORD

Outline all caries and restorations on chart.
Shade in restorations only. See code below.

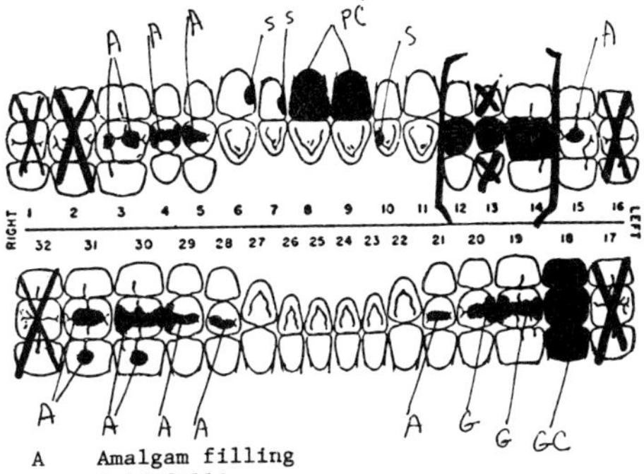

A Amalgam filling
G Gold filling
S Silicate or plastic filling
X Tooth missing
LPM Lost postmortem
PC Porcelain crown
GC Gold crown
SC Steel crown
VC Veneer crown
B Fixed bridge (use brackets beginning and ending with supporting teeth)
PD Partial denture
FD Full denture

Police Case No. H-73-1262
M. E. Case No. H-73-813
City Hartford Date 5 Sept 73

Circumstances requiring examination:
One car accident on I91 in Hartford resulting in fire. Body burned beyond recognition

Site of examination:
University-McCook Hospital, Hartford

Jaw Relationship
- [X] Normal
- [ ] Protruding upper jaw
- [ ] Protruding lower jaw

Prosthetic Appliances
Maxilla
- [X] Fixed Bridge
- [ ] Partial Denture
- [ ] Full Denture

Mandible
- [ ] Fixed Bridge
- [ ] Partial Denture
- [ ] Full Denture

Describe prosthetic appliances:
Veneer crowns on #12 and #14
Cast gold veneer pontic #13

This box to be filled in if identification is made. Date 9 Sept 1973 Time 1415
Name of Deceased Harry S. Murphy
Street and No. 721 Colvin Avenue
City Kenmore State N.Y.
Birthdate 17 Jan 1924 Age 49
Sex Male Race Cauc.

Abnormalities and other oral conditions:
Torus palatinus

Postmortem dental photographs Yes [X] No [ ]
Postmortem dental x-rays Yes [X] No [ ]

Antemortem records obtained from
Name Dr. Stanley H. Wohlfeld
Street and No. 2912 Delaware Ave.
City Kenmore
State New York 14217
Area Code 716 Tel. 876-7400

Name and Address of Examiner:
Dr. Lester L. Luntz
111 Pearl Street
Hartford, Conn. 06103

Describe antemortem records:
Full mouth and bite-wing x-rays
Written treatment charts

Dr. Lester L. Luntz
Signature of Examiner

Officer George Smith, #86, H.P.D.
Name of Investigating Officer

Additional notes on back Yes [ ] No [X]

SP-144-C Rev. 1972

B

No., M.E. (Medical Examiner) Case No. and, possibly, an ID (Bureau of Identification) No. that can be added to the upper right corner of the form. Note anatomical diagram of the dentition in upper left corner and use of Universal numbering system to designate the teeth (see Fig. 5-9). Teeth lost postmortem should be so marked on the chart. No special marking, other than an *X*, is needed to indicate teeth lost antemortem. Provision is made for recording of additional information on reverse side of sheet in the unusual case where it might be necessary. *B*, Example of completed Dental Identification Record.

important to determine whether a tooth was lost antemortem or postmortem (see Chapter 4); adding the letters *LPM* would indicate a tooth lost postmortem. Unerupted teeth, including impacted third molars, should be marked as missing. Partially impacted third molars should also be noted. Teeth present in the dentition and free of pathology remain unmarked on the chart.

Care should be taken to detect teeth that may have shifted position: If the deceased lost the first molar early in life (about 6 to 9 years of age), the second and third molars may have migrated, so that the second molar may occupy the place of the first molar—a situation that could be doubly complicated to discern because, occasionally, the maxillary second molar has the anatomical appearance of the first molar—and the third molar may have moved into the space vacated by the second molar. The cusp of Carabelli, an extra cusp frequently found on the mesial lingual surface of the maxillary first molar, acts as a clue to the presence of the first molar in the dentition. Similarly, confusion can occur where the upper second bicuspid has shifted into the space left by an extracted first bicuspid, especially since in the maxilla the second bicuspid can resemble the first bicuspid and vice versa.

Restorations

Restored teeth and the restorative materials used should be recorded. All restorations should be drawn anatomically, showing shape and size, on the tooth surface involved. Shading in the drawing differentiates it from untreated caries.

To indicate the tooth surface involved, the following code symbols can be used:

M—mesial, surface toward the midline
D—distal, surface away from the midline
F—facial, surface toward the cheek or lip, used instead of buccal (cheek) and labial (lip)
L—lingual, surface toward the tongue
O—occlusal, chewing surface of molar and bicuspid teeth
I—incisal, biting surface of anterior teeth

When more than one surface is involved, a combination of letters is used, for example:

MO—mesial occlusal surfaces
DOF—distal occlusal facial surfaces

Caries

Unshaded outline drawings on the diagrammatic surfaces of the teeth indicate carious lesions (decay) found in the mouth at the time of the postmortem examination. The above code is also used to indicate the location on the tooth of carious lesions and other conditions.

Prostheses

Any prosthetic appliance—fixed bridgework, partial denture, full denture—worn by the deceased at the time of death should be described in detail. Following are guides to general procedures for postmortem charting of prosthetic aids:

Fixed Bridgework. The pontics (dummy teeth), type of abutments (support for the bridge) and overall construction of the bridge should be noted (Fig. 5-5*B*).

1. *Pontics.* Label each pontic as such on the diagrammatic chart. Because pontics replace missing teeth, they should also be marked with an *X*.
2. *Abutments.* Draw abutments (inlays, $^3/_4$ crowns, full crowns, etc.) anatomically on the diagrammatic chart and label.
3. *Construction.* Explain the construction of the bridgework, describing the abutments, pontics (soldered back, cast back, interchangeable, etc.), and any other features.

Partial Denture. If there is a partial (removable) denture

1. Name denture teeth and their material (plastic or porcelain).
2. Name the clasped natural teeth.
3. Describe denture base material (chrome cobalt, gold, acrylic, etc.) and design (lingual bar, web bar, horseshoe, etc.).
4. Indicate evidence of any repairs and additions.
5. Note any unrepaired damage to denture, such as cracks, chipped teeth, or a broken clasp.

Full Dentures. The dentures of a victim often yield many points of information useful to the forensic dentist for making an identification. This is especially true for the anterior maxillary denture teeth, which are structured from a greater variety of shapes and sizes than the other teeth in a denture. Attempting to ascertain specific facts relating to the construction of the denture base and teeth may require painstaking effort; hence, being able to enlist the assistance of a qualified denture technician can be invaluable.

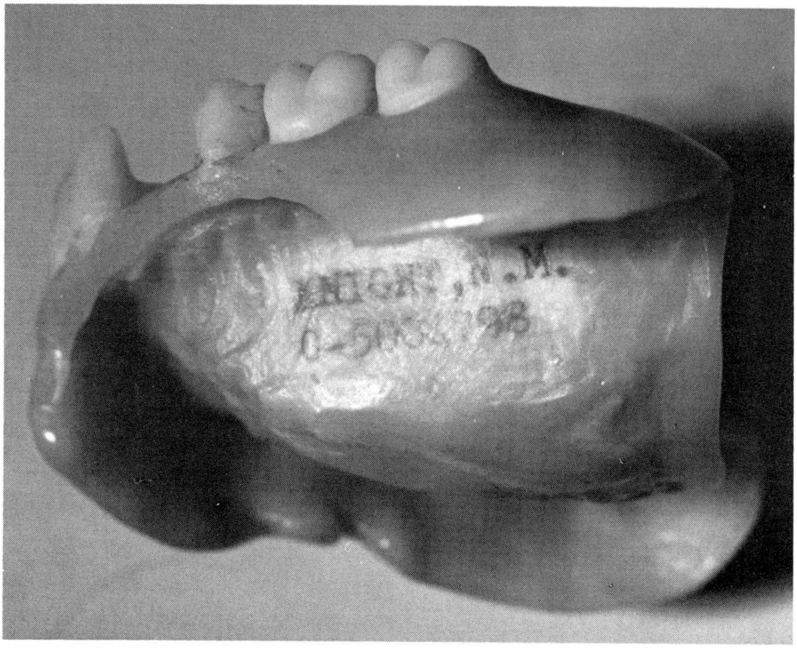

Fig. 5-6. Full denture found with skeletal remains. Victim's name and Veterans Administration claim number had been processed into upper and lower dentures on tissue side, enabling an immediate identification to be made.

1. *Denture Base*

PROCESSED IDENTIFIERS. The tissue side of the denture should be inspected for a name and an identifying number that might have been processed into the denture, a practice frequently followed by military and government agencies (Fig. 5-6).

MATERIAL. The dentist should determine, if possible, the denture base material (acrylic, vinyl, styrene, etc.) and describe it (mottled, veined, darkly pigmented, etc.).

SPECIAL CHARACTERISTICS. Special characteristics to be recorded include deep festooning, post dam, palatal relief (air chamber), rugae, clear palate and characterization.

ALTERATIONS. Note evidence of rebase and any repairs. Describe any damage, such as cracks or breaks.

2. *Denture Teeth*

MANUFACTURER. If ascertainable, the name of the manufacturer should be included in the postmortem record. Companies that pro-

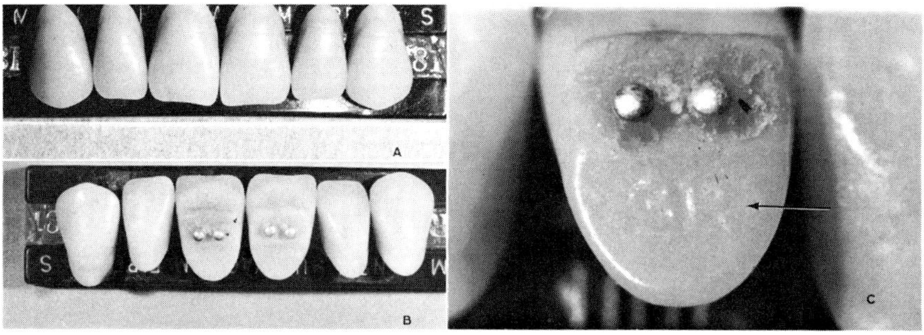

Fig. 5-7. A, Maxillary anterior denture teeth on manufacturer's stick. Denture teeth are produced in a variety of shapes and sizes, classified by mold numbers individual to each manufacturer. *B,* The two first incisors have been reversed on the stick, showing the small, gold pins that retain a porcelain tooth in a denture base. Usually found on this side of a tooth are the mold number and manufacturer's trademark. *C,* The mold number 3*R* on the ridge lap of the tooth (*arrow*) is the manufacturer's designation for this particular shape and size of tooth.

duce denture teeth often put their trademark on the lingual surface (tongue side) of the tooth (e.g., Dentsply teeth have a crescent, Universal teeth a pentagon and Myerson teeth the letter *M*).

MATERIAL. Indicate whether the teeth are made of acrylic (plastic) or porcelain.

MOLD NUMBER. The shapes and sizes of denture teeth are classified by mold numbers, individual to each manufacturer, that frequently appear on the ridge lap of the teeth (Fig. 5-7). To find the mold number on an anterior porcelain tooth in a denture, briefly heat the facial surface of the tooth with a pinpoint flame until the tooth can be removed with a heated spatula from the denture base. The mold number will then, usually, be visible on the ridge lap, if it has not previously been ground. This process cannot be used with acrylic teeth because the ridge lap has usually been ground for retention, thereby removing the mold number. For acrylic and porcelain teeth, where the mold number is not ascertainable from the ridge lap, the shape and size of the tooth should be matched against the manufacturer's mold guide in an effort to derive the mold number.

SHADE NUMBER. With the aid of the manufacturer's shade guide, determine the shade number of the anterior teeth.

POSTERIOR TEETH. Note the type of posterior teeth used in a denture: 33°, 20°, 0° (flat plane), etc.

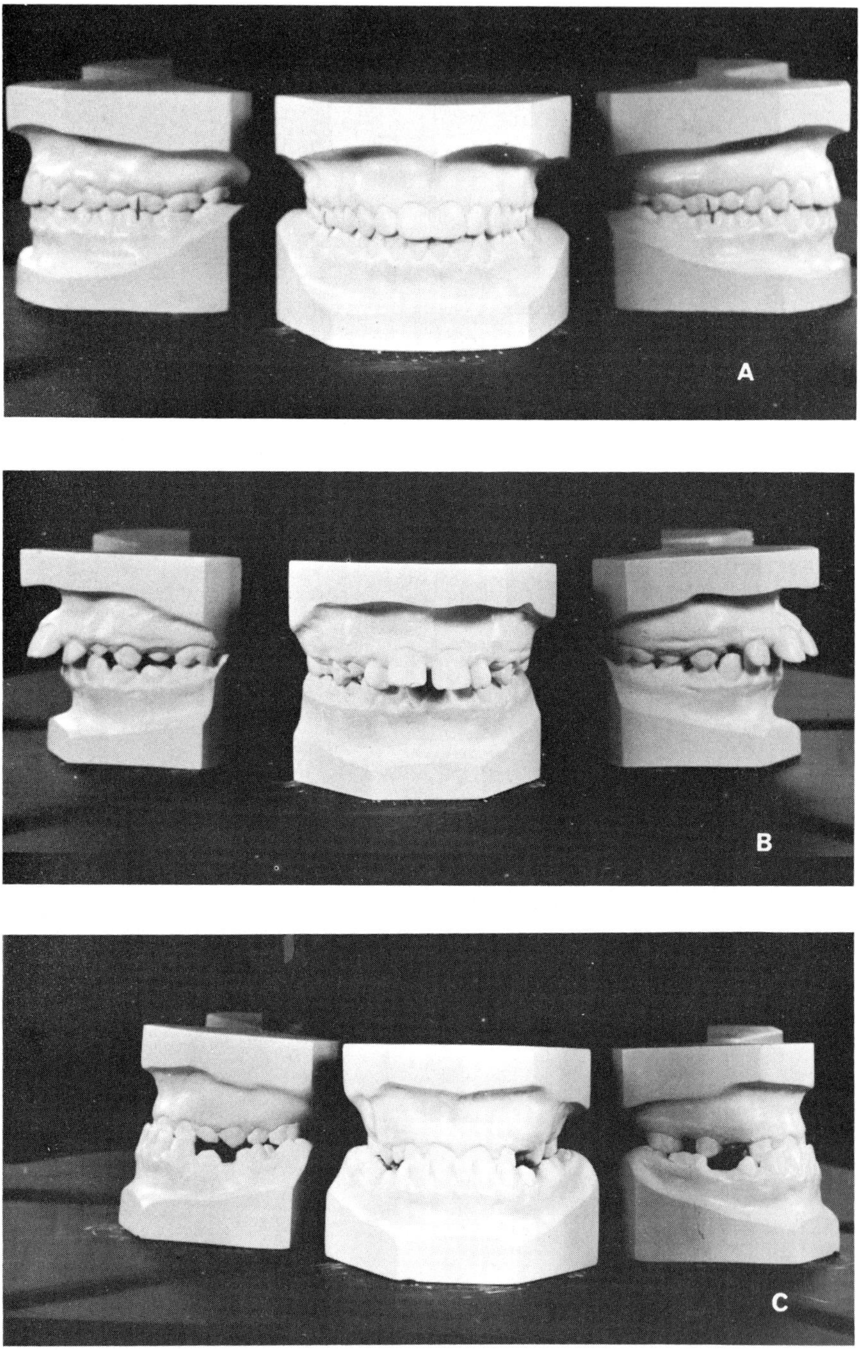

Fig. 5-8. Three-sided views of models, showing jaw relationships. *A,* Teeth with normal occulsion. *B,* Protrusive maxillary anterior teeth. *C,* Protrusive mandibular anterior teeth.

SPECIAL CHARACTERISTICS. Record any special characteristics, e.g., unusual alignment or spacing of the teeth or an unusual set-up (less than fourteen teeth in the denture).

ALTERATIONS. Describe any damage, such as fractured or cracked teeth.

Occlusal Relationship

The occlusal relationship of the jaws can be described by one of the following

1. Normal
2. Protruding upper jaw
3. Protruding lower jaw

Since the dentist in general practice has little occasion to record occlusal relationship, it is likely that the information will be furnished by family or friends of the deceased in lay terms, hence the simplistic terminology employed here (Fig. 5-8).

Anomalies

Any unusual conditions in the oral cavity should be recorded, such as

1. Diastema—an unnatural space between two teeth
2. Rotated tooth—a tooth turned in its socket
3. Unusual tooth formation—extra cusps, pegshaped incisors, fused teeth, hypoplasia, etc.
4. Unusual wear facets of teeth—abnormal wear patterns evidenced on the teeth of the pipe smoker, bobby pin opener, nail-clenching carpenter, tack-holding upholsterer and others.
5. Abnormal pigmentation in tooth structure
6. Unusual tooth alignment
7. Lesions in the soft tissue
8. Abnormal gingival pigmentation
9. Torus palatinus—bony growth found in palate of maxilla
10. Torus mandibularis—bony growth found unilaterally or bilaterally on lingual surface of mandible
11. Defects in maxilla or mandible—cleft palate, excessive bone loss in edentulous areas, oversized tuberosities, etc.

Age Estimation

Although the average dentist called upon to assist in identification does not have sophisticated scientific equipment at his disposal or, generally speaking, the expertise for using it, there are a few broad guidelines that he can employ, at times, to estimate the age of the deceased:

1. Extensive wear on teeth usually does not appear on a person under age 50.
2. Excessive bone loss usually does not occur under age 40.
3. Closure of the third molar root apex usually does not occur before the age of 20.
4. For estimating age under 13, the Schour and Massler chart "Development of the Human Dentition," available from the American Dental Association, is fairly reliable—within a margin of six months to a year.

However, since age ascertainment through dental indicants is not an exact science, a statement of age would not be included on the Dental Identification Record unless specifically requested by the investigating agency.

THE UNIVERSAL SYSTEM

Attempts to eliminate the complications and confusion caused by the many different systems of dental notation in use throughout the world and to establish a uniform method of dental charting have not succeeded. Yet acceptance by dentists of a standardized system of charting has never been more relevant than at present—in a populous world characterized by ever-swifter international travel, almost instantaneous communication, and imminent computerized conformity. Surely it must seem paradoxical that modern dentists, practicing in the same town—even in the same professional building—may be using dissimilar methods for charting the mouth. The implications are apparent when one contemplates the inevitable increase in mass disasters, the resultant need for prompt record transmission with minimal errors and misconceptions and the arduous task of reviewing and comparing diverse dental records.

One of the most widely used methods in the United States for designating the teeth is known as the Universal System (1–16, 17–32). Now commonly taught in American dental schools, it has been adopted by the Armed Forces, U.S. government agencies (U.S. Public Health Service, Veteran's Administration, etc.), insurance companies and dental organizations. Based on the simple schema of each tooth being assigned its own number (Fig. 5-9), the Universal System

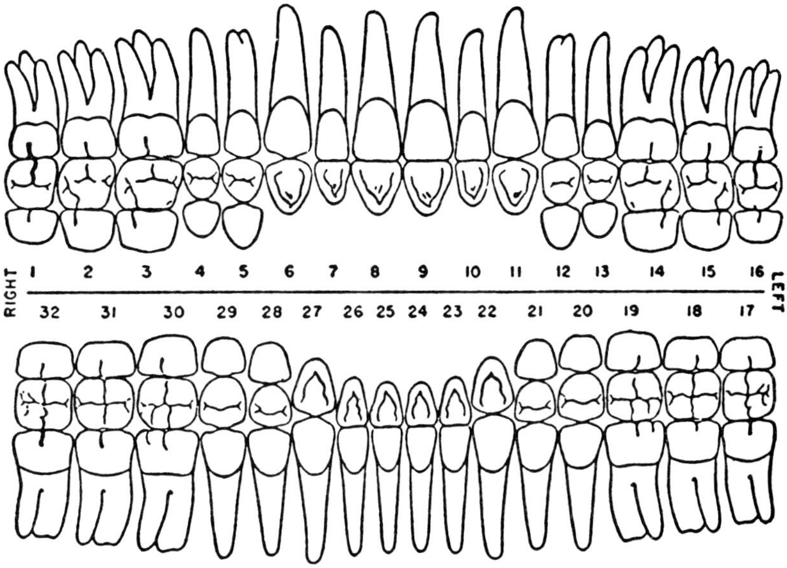

Fig. 5-9. In the Universal System, which is one of the most widely accepted methods in the United States for designating the teeth, each tooth in the mouth has been assigned a specific number (from 1 to 32), starting with the patient's upper right third molar and moving consecutively from right to left, then dropping directly below to the lower left third molar (No. 17) and moving, this time, from left to right. The designations of "right" and "left" on the diagrammatic chart refer to the right- and left-hand sides of the patient. Since the chart is used from the dentist's viewpoint as he faces the patient, the right-hand side of the chart represents the left side of the patient's mouth and vice versa.

The listing below supplies the dental nomenclature for each tooth in the mouth, corresponding to the number on the chart. The vernacular name is given in parentheses.

	Tooth Number	*Nomenclature*
Maxilla	1	Upper right third molar (wisdom tooth)
	2	Upper right second molar (twelve-year molar)
	3	Upper right first molar (six-year molar)
	4	Upper right second bicuspid or second premolar
	5	Upper right first bicuspid or first premolar
	6	Upper right cuspid or canine (eyetooth)
	7	Upper right second incisor or lateral incisor
	8	Upper right first incisor or central incisor
	9	Upper left first incisor or central incisor
	10	Upper left second incisor or lateral incisor
	11	Upper left cuspid or canine (eyetooth)

	Tooth Number	*Nomenclature*	*Tooth Number*	*Nomenclature*
	12	Upper left first bicuspid or first premolar	23	Lower left second incisor or lateral incisor
	13	Upper left second bicuspid or second premolar	24	Lower left first incisor or central incisor
	14	Upper left first molar (six-year molar)	25	Lower right first incisor or central incisor
	15	Upper left second molar (twelve-year molar)	26	Lower right second incisor or lateral incisor
	16	Upper left third molar (wisdom tooth)	27	Lower right cuspid or canine
Mandible	17	Lower left third molar (wisdom tooth)	28	Lower right first bicuspid or first premolar
	18	Lower left second molar (twelve-year molar)	29	Lower right second bicuspid or second premolar
	19	Lower left first molar (six-year molar)	30	Lower right first molar (six-year molar)
	20	Lower left second bicuspid or second premolar	31	Lower right second molar (twelve-year molar)
	21	Lower left first bicuspid or first premolar	32	Lower right third molar (wisdom tooth)
	22	Lower left cuspid or canine		

satisfies several requirements: It is readily learned, easy to use and quickly comprehended on a diagrammatic chart. In addition, it can be typewritten and lends itself to being transmitted and computerized. For these reasons and in view of its extensive acceptance, the Universal System is the method of choice for postmortem dental charting.

6 X-ray Techniques in Dental Identification

Because of its accuracy, the dental x-ray is the most desirable antemortem record for use in dental identification. The most reliable data upon which to base a dental identification are derived from a comparison of the antemortem and postmortem x-rays. Since it can be assumed that dentists are already acquainted with the general principles of x-raying as applied to positioning the film, angulation, exposure time and processing, only x-ray techniques pertaining to dental identification will be discussed here.

Although the regular x-ray machine in the dental office can be used for postmortem roentgenograms, the problem remains of getting the subject to the office. There is not likely to be an x-ray machine in the morgue. Moreover, even in a hospital the dentist may encounter difficulty obtaining postmortem x-rays. Hospital personnel are often reluctant to cooperate because of the particular problems involved: odors, the possibility of contamination and general difficulty in handling the subject for dental roentgenograms.

Fortunately, the problem can be solved by taking the portable Min-X-Ray machine to the site of the postmortem dental examination. Other x-ray devices are available, such as the Iodine 125 pen, but in view of their cost and restricted usability, they are generally not feasible for postmortem dental x-rays. The equipment for postmortem dental roentgenology (i.e., the Min-X-Ray; the Uni-Chem Single Solution System, a portable x-ray developing kit, and the ruby bulb safelight) are described in Chapter 3.

TAKING POSTMORTEM DENTAL X-RAYS

The techniques employed in taking postmortem dental x-rays differ from those used for antemortem x-rays in the following aspects:

1. Exposure time
2. Positioning and supporting the head or dentition
3. Positioning and supporting the film

Before commencing to x-ray, the forensic dentist should survey the room to see that all personnel, loaded cameras and film are out of the range of radiation. Accidental exposure to radiation will fog photographic and x-ray film.

Exposure Time

To x-ray the jaw of a deceased, a reduction of approximately one-third to one-half the normal exposure time may be required, depending on the thickness of the tissue being x-rayed. The initial roentgenogram, serving as a trial exposure, should be developed immediately. Using that as a basis, the dentist can make any necessary adjustments, increasing or decreasing the exposure time accordingly.

Skeletonized Jaw. To x-ray the skeletonized jaw requires about one-half the exposure time as the normal jaw in a living or deceased person.

Nonskeletonized Jaw. To x-ray a jaw where a partial loss of soft tissue has occurred, for instance, through decomposition, incineration, or resection, requires about two-thirds the normal exposure time.

Positioning and Supporting the Head or Dentition

When the dentition is x-rayed postmortem, a careful attempt should be made to place it in the same position seen in the antemortem x-ray, so that the postmortem x-ray will, so far as possible, duplicate the antemortem film.

Skeletonized or Resected Jaw. The usual dental angulations are used when a resected jaw or detached, skeletonized head is x-rayed, since the dentition can be positioned like that in the normal, living patient, that is, with the plane of occlusion parallel to the floor. Modeling clay can be used to support the jaws or head for x-rays and, sometimes, for photographs as well.

Nonskeletonized Jaw. When the jaws are intact in a nonskeletonized, supine body, it is necessary to adjust the angulation of the x-ray cone, since the subject is in a horizontal position instead of in the normal, upright position of the living patient.

Positioning and Supporting the Film

For postmortem x-rays the film must be retained in the proper relationship to both the dentition and the head of the x-ray machine. This is achieved by first positioning the film relative to the dentition and then focusing the x-ray cone at the correct angulation to the film (Fig. 6-1). Owing to the danger of radiation, the film should never be hand held by the forensic dentist or anyone assisting him. Where it is difficult to retain the film in position, it may prove helpful to utilize one of the many varieties of commercial film holders available, a few of which are mentioned below. Brief experimentation will probably be necessary to determine the best method, in a particular case, of positioning and supporting the film for a postmortem x-ray.

Bite-Wing Tabs. Affixing one end of a wing tab to the center front surface of a film packet and closing the teeth over the opposite end of the tab will produce a bite-wing x-ray when the film is exposed. If the wing tab is attached to the top edge of the packet and the film is properly positioned in the mouth by means of a hemostat clamped to the free end of the tab and resting on the occlusal surface of the teeth, the resulting exposure will be a periapical x-ray. There are a variety of commercial bite-wing tabs on the market that work, more or less, as described here, one of which is Sta-put Bite-wing Tabs ($1.85 per hundred).*

Although not as convenient to use for supporting a film packet as a commercial bite-wing tab, a two-inch piece of transparent, adhesive cellulose tape can be converted into a bite-wing tab by folding the tape in half, with the adhesive sides inward, and sticking it together from the crease to halfway back on itself. If the open legs at the end opposite the crease are stuck to the center front surface of a film packet and the creased end of the tab is placed between the teeth, a bite-wing x-ray will be produced when the film is exposed. If the tab is attached to the top edge of a film packet, it will result in a periapical x-ray. As with commercial bite-wing tabs, a hemostat clamped to the creased edge of the cellulose tape and resting on the occlusal surface of the teeth will retain the film in

* D-P Company, Glendale, California.

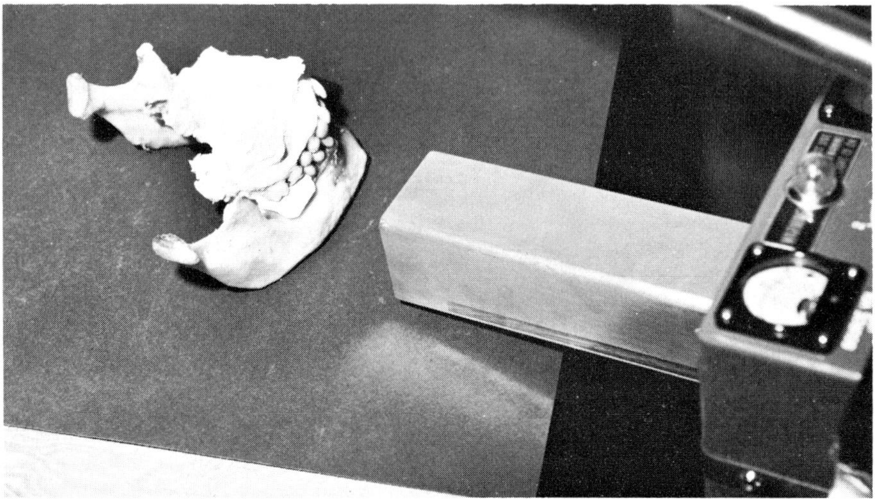

Fig. 6-1. Bite-wing film positioned in jaws for postmortem x-ray.

position for the periapical exposure. In some cases it is possible that a hemostat clamped directly to the edge of a film packet will be the only support needed.

*Stabe Film Holder.** A disposable dental x-ray holder ($7.95 per hundred) made of polystyrene, the Stabe film holder is easily impressed on the occlusal surface of the teeth, thereby retaining the film in position for the x-ray (Fig. 6-2).

Snap-A-Ray Film Holder.† A nondisposable plastic film holder $3 apiece) usable for most exposures and angulations where the head is intact, the Snap-A-Ray (Fig. 6-3) can go into cold sterilization for reuse.

Premier Angulator.‡ The Premier Angulator ($4.50) is a nondisposable nylon film holder (Fig. 6-4), which can be sterilized by autoclaving, boiling or cold chemicals. It is useful when the head is intact.

Modeling Clay. When modeling clay is utilized to hold the x-ray film in a dry skeletonized head (Fig. 6-5), care should be taken to see that there is no clay in front of the film to block the exposure.

* Greene Dental Products, Inc., San Fernando, California.
† Rinn Corp., Elgin, Illinois.
‡ Premier Dental Products, Philadelphia, Pennsylvania.

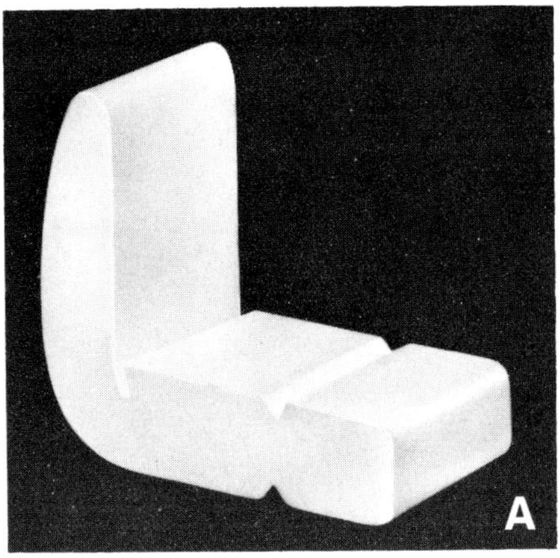

Fig. 6-2. A, Stabe film holder (Courtesy of Greene Dental Products, Inc.); *B,* used to retain x-ray film in correct position in mandible.

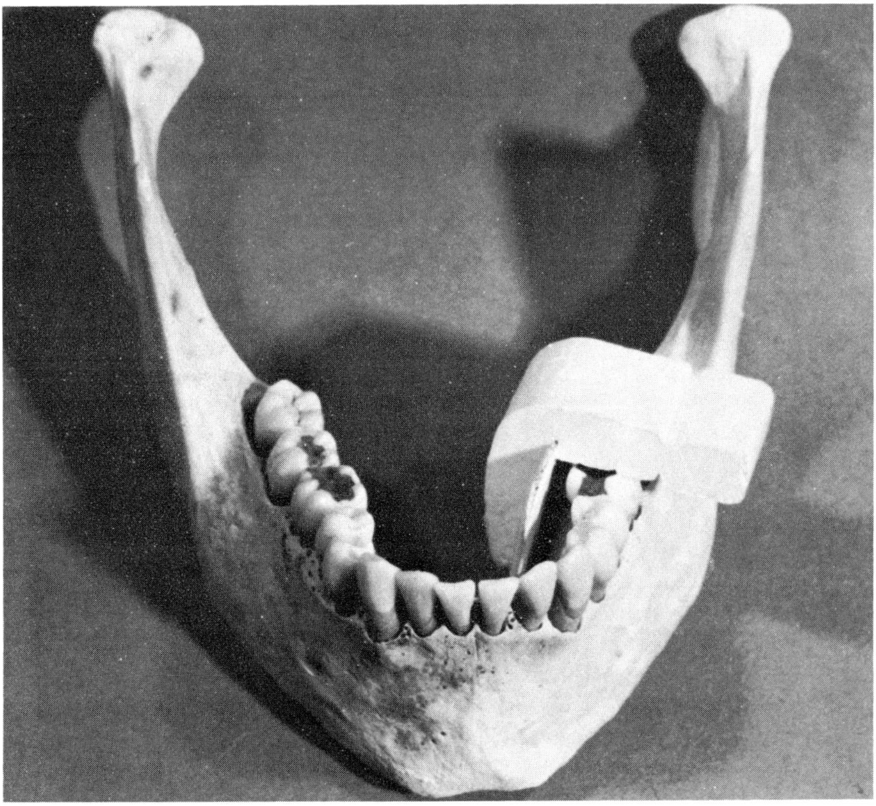

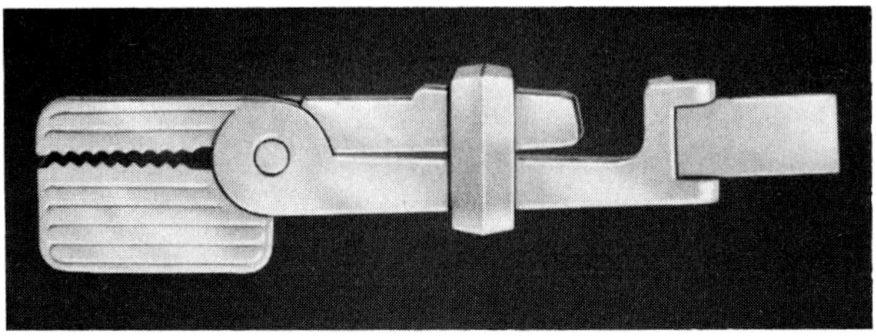

Fig. 6-3. Close-up of Snap-A-Ray film holder. (Courtesy of Rinn Corp.)

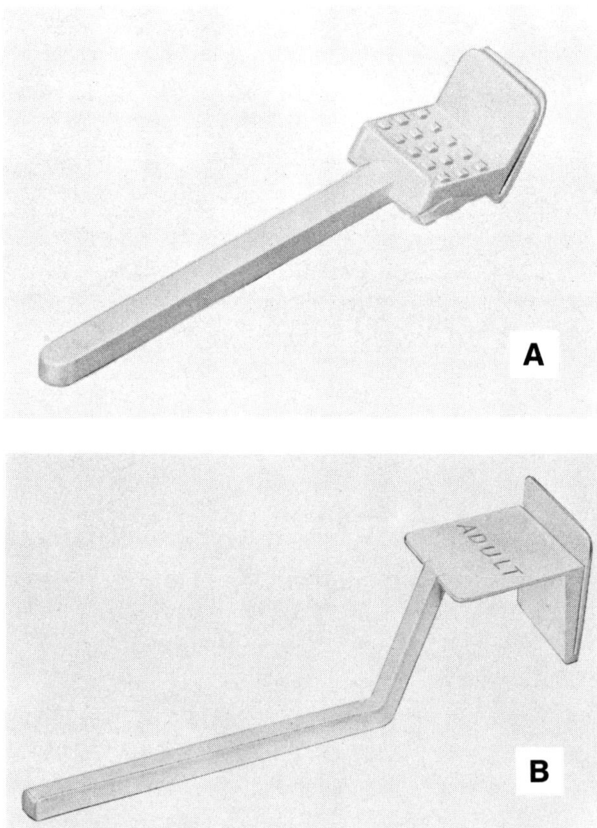

Fig. 6-4. The Premier Angulator film holder. *A,* Model used for periapicals. *B,* Model used for bite-wings. (Photographs courtesy of Premier Dental Products Company)

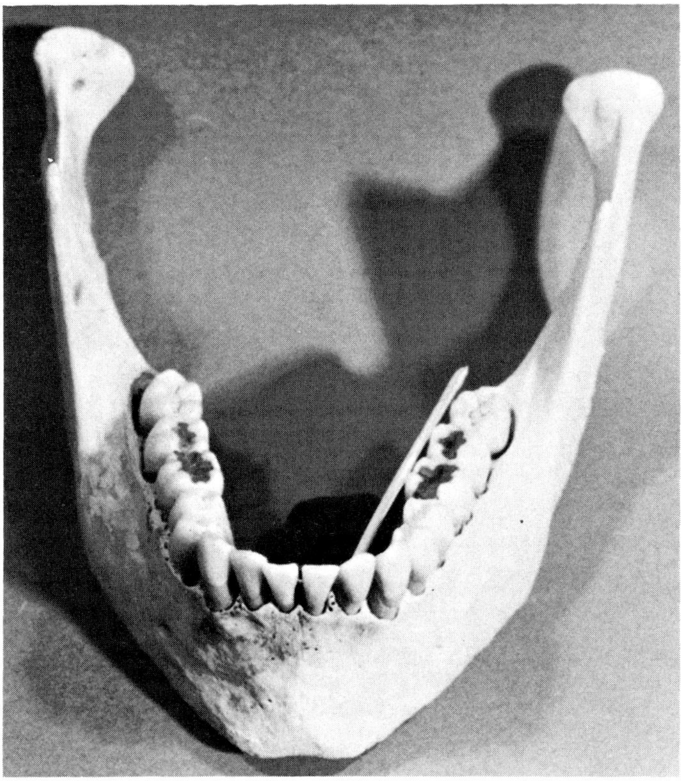

Fig. 6-5. Modeling clay used to support x-ray film in dry skeletonized jaw.

DUPLICATING X-RAYS

In those instances where the dentist has requested the return of his antemortem records, the antemortem x-rays should be duplicated before they are sent back. When a dental darkroom is used for duplicating x-rays, the additional items needed are duplicating film, a photographic printing frame or similar device, stopwatch and film hanger for 8 × 10-inch film (Fig. 6-6). The duplication of x-rays is a simple but important technique, useful not only in dental identification but for educational and consultative purposes as well.

Equipment

1. Kodak RP/D X-Omat Radiograph Duplicating Film, 8 × 10 inches ($19.80 for fifty sheets)

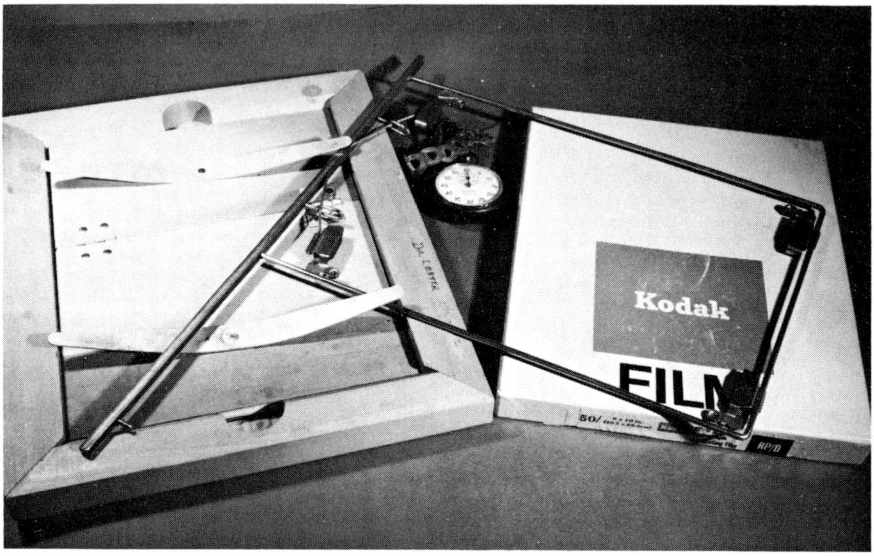

Fig. 6-6. The additional items needed in a dental darkroom to duplicate x-rays are photographic printing frame, film hanger, stopwatch and duplicating film.

2. 15-watt safelight with Kodak Safelight Filter No. 6B (brown) or ML-2 (light orange)
3. Kodak Dental X-ray Developer and Fixer (for manual processing)
4. Photographic printing frame, 8 × 10 inches (about $6.25)
5. Film hanger for 8 × 10-inch film ($10.50)
6. Stopwatch

The above items can be obtained from a dental supply company, with the exception of the printing frame, which is sold in photography stores.

Procedure

Kodak Radiograph Duplicating Film makes duplicate x-rays directly from the originals by exposure to tungsten, daylight fluorescent or ultraviolet light. In the darkroom, at a distance of four feet or more from the safelight, the film can be handled before and after exposure and during processing. Care should be taken to avoid leaving fingermarks or otherwise marring the film. The following steps for duplicating x-rays are performed in the darkroom under the safelight:

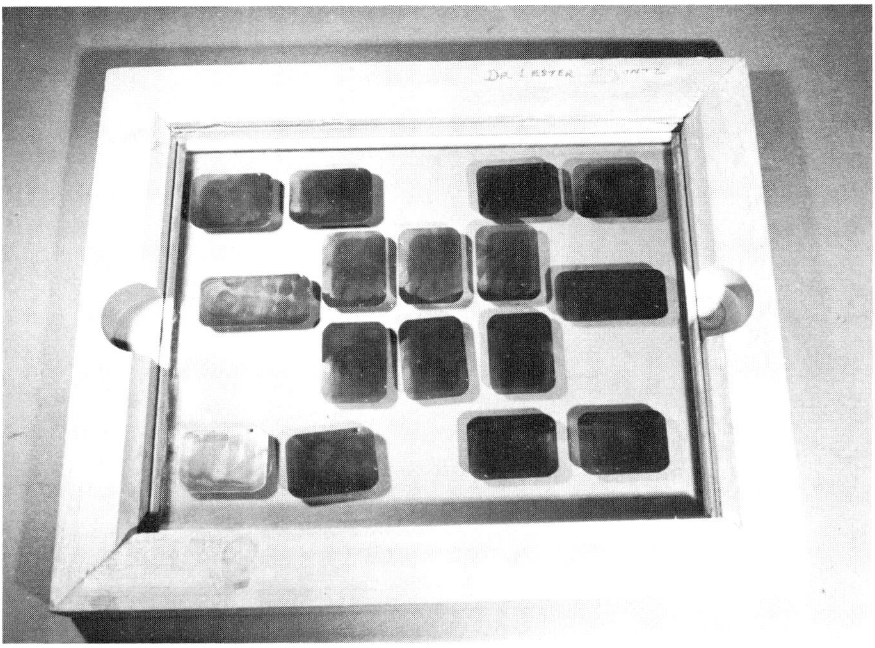

Fig. 6-7. X-rays should be positioned in the printing frame according to the order desired in the duplicate film.

1. Place printing frame with the glass side down and remove the tension-spring back. On the inner side of the glass, in the frame, position the x-rays that are to be duplicated (Fig. 6-7).
2. Remove a sheet of duplicating film from the light-tight box, reclosing immediately to shield the remaining films from exposure. If desired, the 8 × 10-inch film sheet, which is the smallest available size, can be cut into smaller sizes.
3. Place the light color emulsion side of the duplicating film directly over the radiographs on the glass (Fig. 6-8).
4. Replace the tension-spring back of the printing frame to maintain direct contact between the radiographs and the duplicating film. This also serves to retain the x-rays in position when the frame is inverted (Fig. 6-9).
5. Invert the frame so that the glass side now faces the light source (Fig. 6-10). With a stopwatch or second sweep hand to gauge the time, a trial exposure should be made at twenty seconds or thereabouts, depending upon the light source. Increased exposure time lightens the picture tone. Contrast can be heightened by varying the

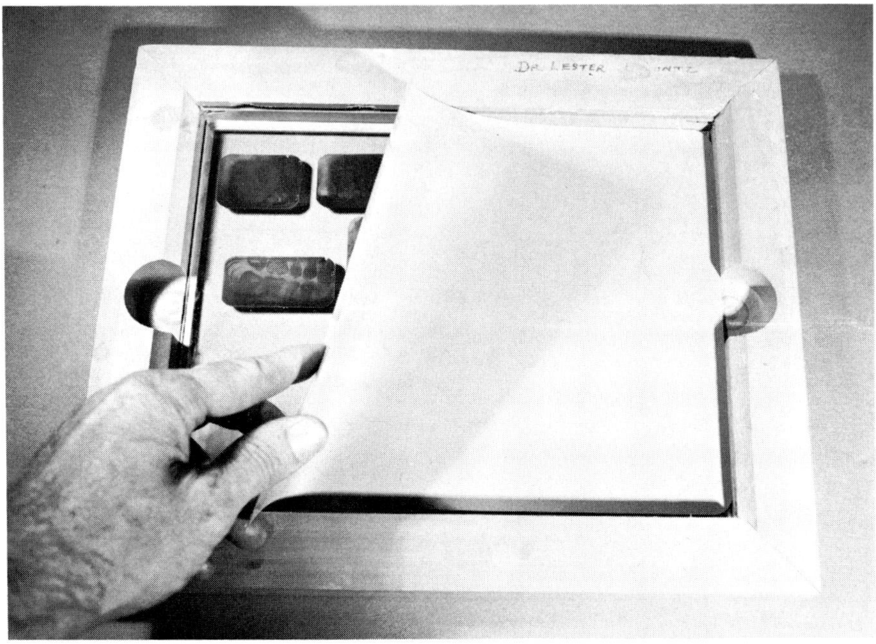

Fig. 6-8. The emulsion side of the film is placed in contact with the x-rays.

intensity of the light or by using whiter light. With such adjustments it is possible for the quality of the original radiograph to be improved upon in the duplicate.

6. After exposure, the duplicating film is removed from the frame and clipped to the film hanger (Fig. 6-11). Standard darkroom techniques are employed to develop the film manually with Kodak Dental X-ray Developer, according to the time and temperature instructions. Then fix, wash and dry the film.

For rapid, automatic processing, the Kodak RP X-Omat Processor, found in most modern hospitals, processes duplicating film in ninety seconds (Fig. 6-12).

Other Duplicating Techniques

Other techniques for duplicating x-rays either require the use of more sophisticated equipment or produce duplicates of lesser quality than the method described above. However, for the dentist desiring to duplicate merely an x-ray or two on infrequent occasions, the

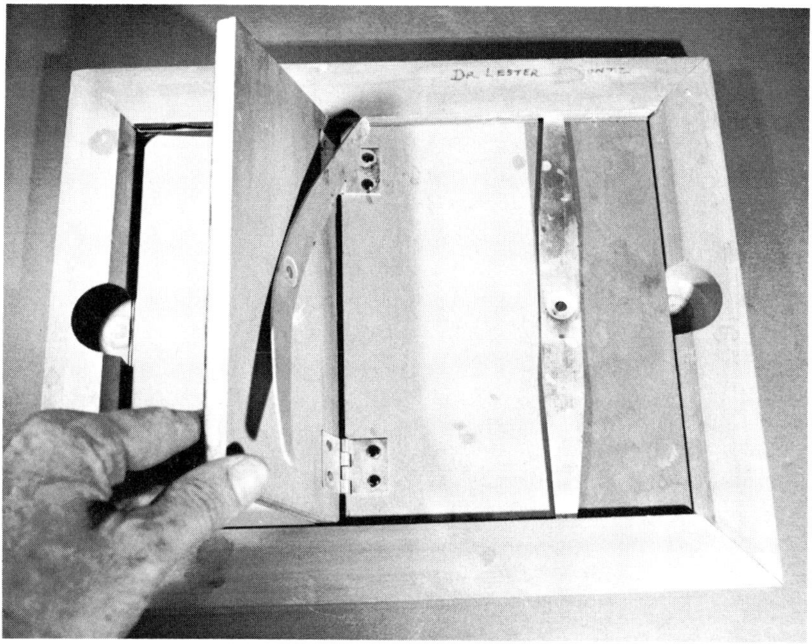

Fig. 6-9. The back of the printing frame retains the duplicating film in tight contact with the x-rays.

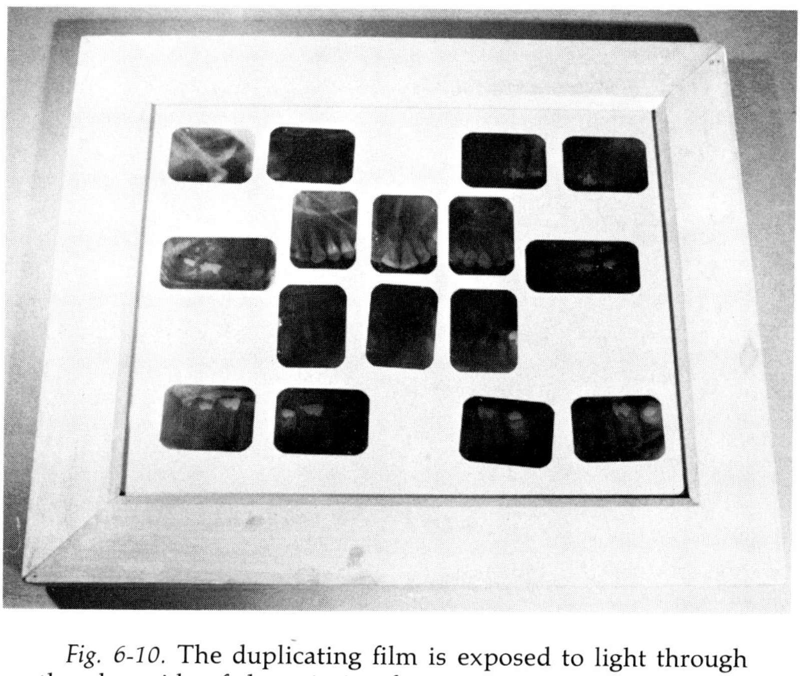

Fig. 6-10. The duplicating film is exposed to light through the glass side of the printing frame.

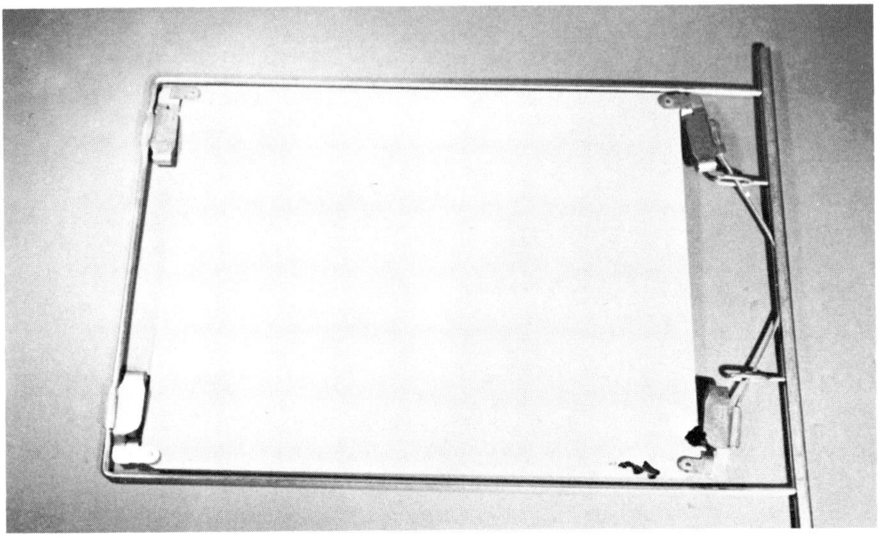

Fig. 6-11. After exposure, the duplicating film is clipped to the film hanger for developing manually.

following simple techniques may serve his purpose without an investment in special duplicating film, a printing frame, or other equipment.

Photographing the X-ray. One or more x-rays atop an x-ray view box can be photographed in color or black-and-white with a 35mm SLR TTL camera and macro lens (see Chapter 7). If a view box is not available, the x-rays can be taped to a window with cellulose tape and photographed with the sky as a light source. The reproduction will not equal the quality obtained when duplicating film is used.

Commercial Duplication of Periapicals. Eastman Kodak duplicates periapical x-rays in the same manner used for duplicating Kodachrome slides. The periapical first must be placed in a 2 × 2-inch cardboard mount and then can be given to a local dealer to be sent to Eastman Kodak for duplication. Probably the main disadvantage is that it takes at least a week for the dentist to receive the duplicate.

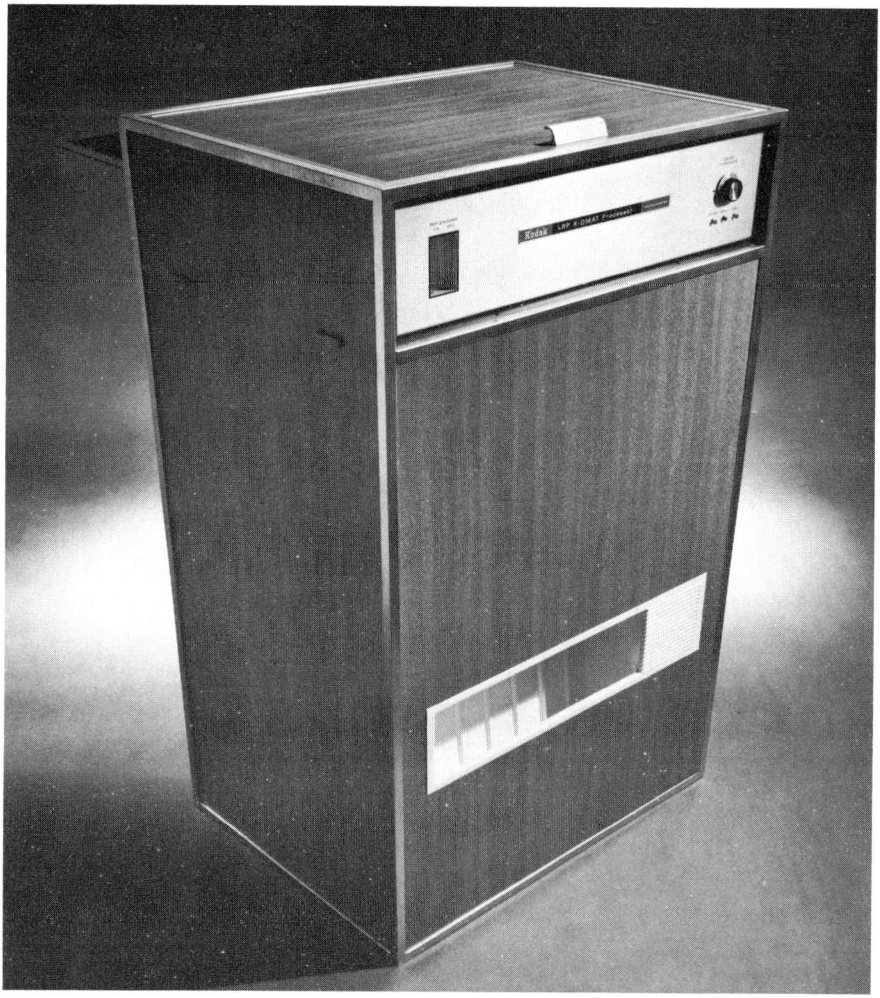

Fig. 6-12. The Kodak RP X-Omat Processor. The exposed duplicating film is inserted into the darkroom side of the machine; ninety seconds later, the processed film is delivered from the opposite side of the machine (*above*), in a normally lit room. (Courtesy of Eastman Kodak Company)

7 Photographic Equipment

"One picture is worth more than ten thousand words" aptly applies to dental identification. The picture does not displace the written record, but is an important adjunct, clarifying and expanding it. Thus, a photographic record, included with written reports, enhances and completes the file on a case.

The advantages of the photographic record are many: Its accuracy and reliability are widely accepted; its clarity and comprehensibility scale language barriers; relationships of size and shape can often be depicted; even a minutiae of details can be rapidly recorded and studied later at length; and as verifiable evidence, its trustworthiness generally goes unquestioned.

Specifically relevant to dental identification, the photograph reveals the outline, size and, sometimes, material of restorations, the contour of individual teeth, form of the arch, design of a partial denture, including the shapes of clasps, and other dental details. Even a scrupulously written report is unlikely to be as graphic as the actual pictorial record, and a succint report may omit certain details. If a dental examination was performed under less than optimal conditions, it is possible for certain details, obscure or unobserved at the time, to be captured in a photograph and later, under careful scrutiny, to become discernible.

Inasmuch as the forensic dentist, unable to predict the precise conditions under which he will be operating, should strive to be self-sufficient and prepared for any eventuality, so is it advisable that he know at least the rudiments of photography for such reasons as: (1) a police officer may not be available to take photographs, (2) a police officer is not likely to be trained in close-up photography or have the specialized equipment and (3) a dentist who takes his own pictures can retain control of all his records, preserving the chain of evidence intact.

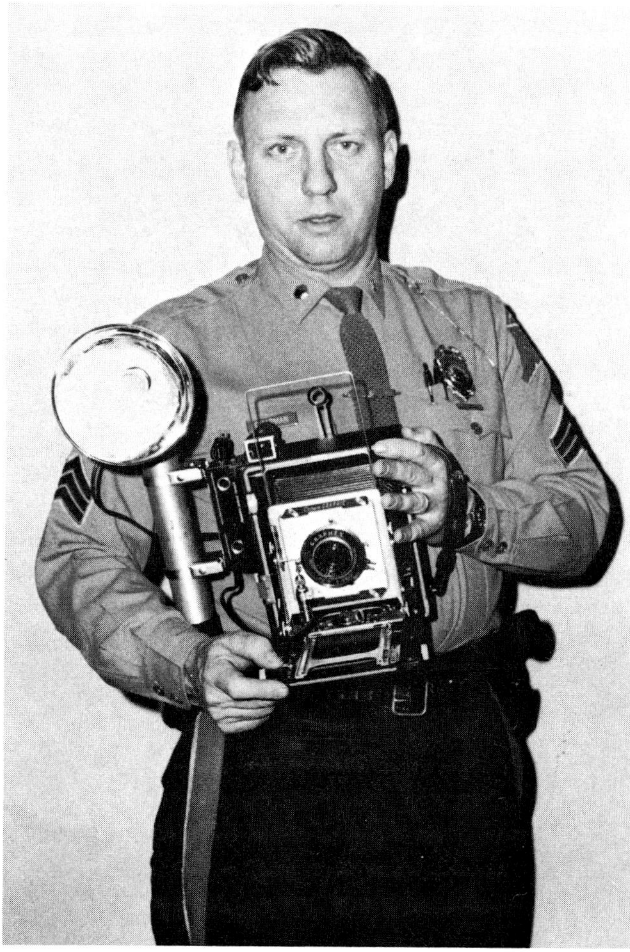

Fig. 7-1. The police officer familiar with photography is a valuable assistant to the forensic dentist. (Connecticut State Police)

PHOTOGRAPHING THE VICTIM

If the police officer assisting the dentist has a knowledge of photography, the officer should be instructed to bring with him a press-type camera and flashbulbs (Fig. 7-1), which may have a side benefit, since they can be used to disperse the maggots often found on a decomposed body during the summer months. Being photosensitive, the

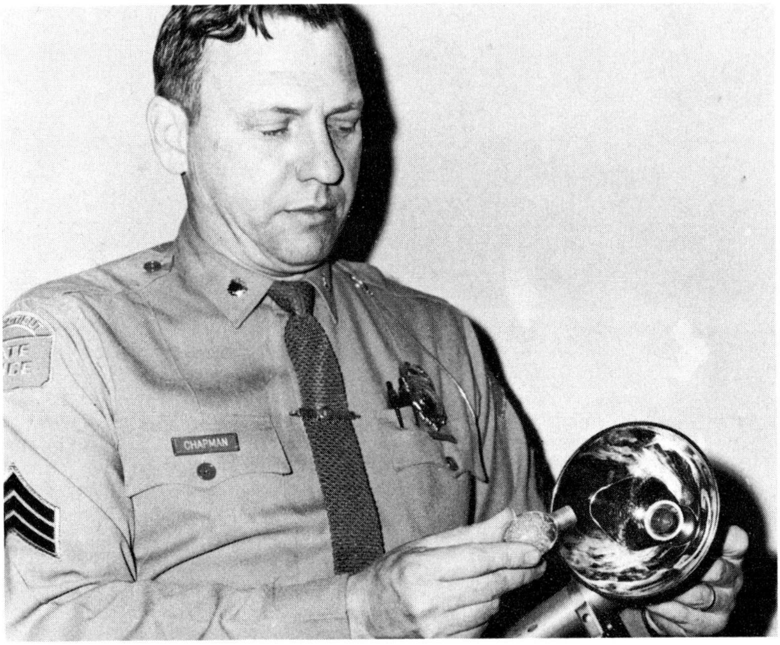

Fig. 7-2. Flashbulbs can be used not only to furnish the photographic light source but also to disperse maggots, which are photosensitive. (Connecticut State Police)

maggots will move off into darker recesses when a few flashbulbs are fired in their direction (Fig. 7-2).

Initially, the head and face of the victim should be photographed in color by the dentist and in color or black-and-white by the police officer, thereby recording the appearance and condition prior to the dental examination and any ensuing facial disturbances. The following color pictures should also be taken: occlusal views of the mandibular and maxillary arches; anterior views of the dentition, including, if possible, the jaws in occlusion, and if the jaws have been resected, lateral views of the dentition to show occlusion. In addition, close-up pictures should be taken of any uncommon dental conditions, such as unusual bridgework, malformed teeth or other anomalies, etc. To support the dry skull or resected jaws for photographs, modeling clay can be used.

Taking several shots of each view eliminates the need to make copies for the medical examiner, police and other interested parties. Shooting with color transparency film, Kodachrome or Ektachrome,

EASTMAN KODAK COMPANY
COLOR PRINT AND PROCESSING SALES AND SERVICE
ROCHESTER 4, NEW YORK

TELEPHONE
GLADSTONE 8-1000

State of New York:
: SS
County of Monroe :

, being duly sworn deposes and says that he is employed as in the Film Processing Laboratory, Kodak Park, of Eastman Kodak Company, Rochester, New York 14650.

That his department received on and processed-

No. of Rolls, Size and Type:

Order Nos:

From Dealer:

Customer:

That the film was not cut, mutilated, or altered in any manner during processing (except that if identified above as "8mm film" it was slit from 16mm width after processing and spliced in accordance with standard operating procedures). That while the film was in the possession of Eastman Kodak Company it was not shown to any person other than employees of said laboratory of known integrity in the ordinary course of handling the same.

Further, that the end of the processed film and the carton flap were perforated by Eastman Kodak Company at the time of processing with the following identification number(s):

and that this film and this affidavit were returned under Kodak seal to

____

Sworn to before me this

_____day of__________________,196_

____

Fig. 7-3. On request, Eastman Kodak will furnish the above affidavit at no charge.

allows the dentist to send the film in mailers by first-class mail directly to Eastman Kodak for processing; Eastman Kodak will return the slides by first-class mail directly to the dentist. This procedure is generally accepted in the United States as maintaining an unbroken chain of evidence (Fig. 7-3). Where copies of a photograph are to be widely distributed for broad publicity, as in the circulation of a release seeking information on an unknown, the photograph should be taken in black-and-white, which is easier and cheaper to duplicate than a color print and, also, is the medium used for publication in newspapers and professional journals.

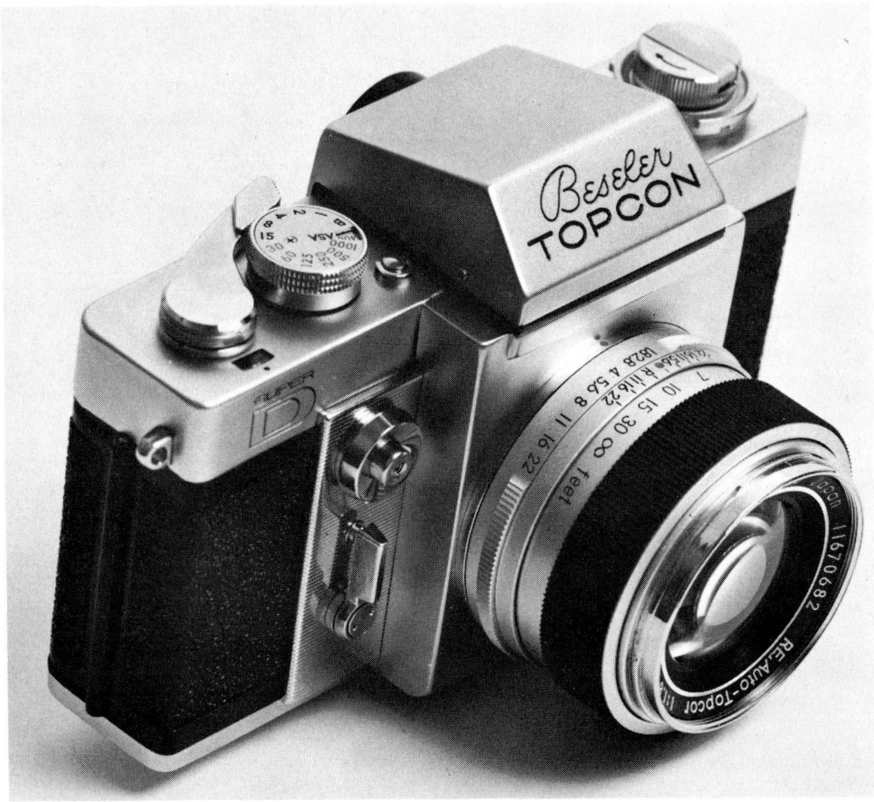

Fig. 7-4. An example of a quality 35mm camera with SLR (single-lens reflex) and TTL (through-the-lens metering). This type of camera is easily adapted to close-up dental photography. (Courtesy of Beseler Topcon)

CLOSE-UP PHOTOGRAPHY

Camera Accessories

Most of the photographs taken in dental identification fall within the realm of close-up photography, that is, the area to be photographed is closer than the minimum distance to which a 35mm camera can be focused, using the normal lens (Fig. 7-4). Ordinarily, the normal lens will focus down to 18 to 22 inches from the subject. Closer focusing entails moving the lens farther out from the camera body or adding plus lenses to the normal lens without extending it. Reversing the lens, using an adapter, has limited usage for close-up work and, therefore, directions for its use are not included here.

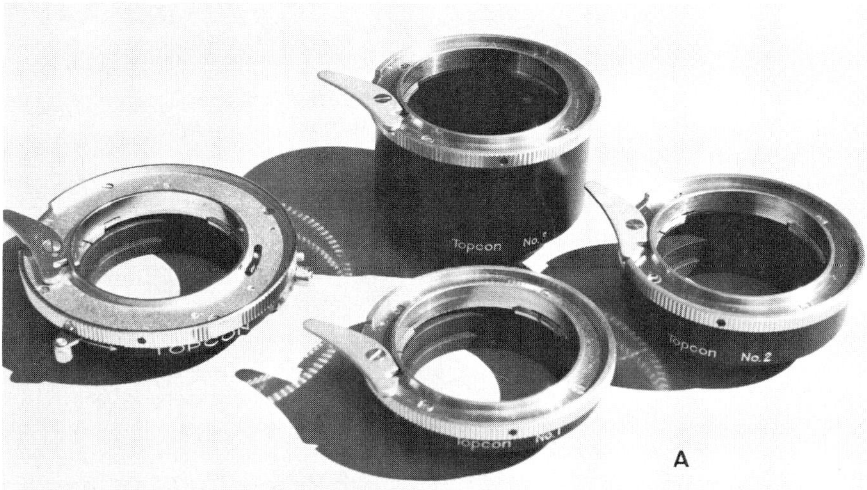

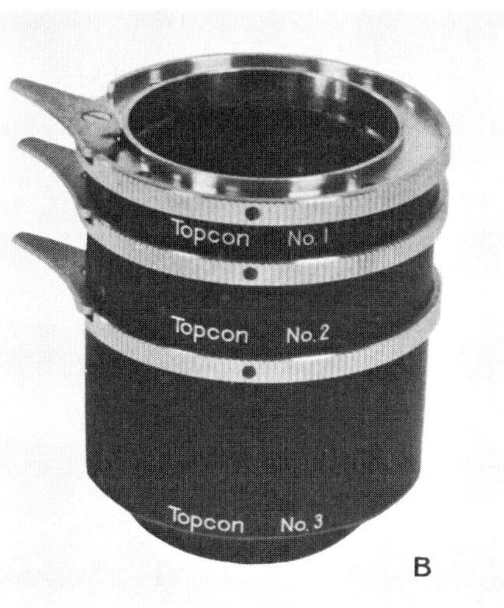

Fig. 7-5. A, Extension tubes of varying lengths. *B,* Using additional extension tubes between the camera and the lens gives greater magnification. (Courtesy of Beseler Topcon)

Extending the Lens

The use of the bellows attachment or extension tubes enables the normal lens to be extended from the camera body for close-ups, producing larger images than can be obtained by using the normal lens alone.

Extension Tubes. Of varying lengths for fixed distances, rigid extension tubes, singly or in various combinations, are attached to the camera body with the lens affixed to the end of the extension tube. The amount of extension between the lens and film plane controls the degree of magnification to be produced in the picture image (Fig. 7-5).

Bellows. The bellows attachment, being more flexible than the rigid extension tubes, provides both greater selection and greater magnification. Modifications are readily made by simply sliding the bellows backward or forward (Fig. 7-6), a less troublesome process than interchanging tubes. However, the bellows does not retract enough to match the minimal magnification of the shortest extension tube. The bellows attachment and extension tubes can also be used conjointly.

Macro Lens. Without the use of accessory devices, the macro lens can be extended farther from the camera body than the normal lens and can be focused from infinity down to about 4 inches. Although the maximal degree of magnification provided is less than that obtainable by using the bellows or extension tubes, the macro lens, its optics having been specifically designed for close-up work, is quite satisfactory for dental photography. Because it is slower and requires more light than the normal lens, the macro lens, generally, is not used in regular photography (Fig. 7-7). It is available for many different makes of 35mm camera, including the Nikon, Nikkormat, Minolta and Topcon.

Magnifying Lenses

The plus (+) lens, procurable for most cameras, offers another

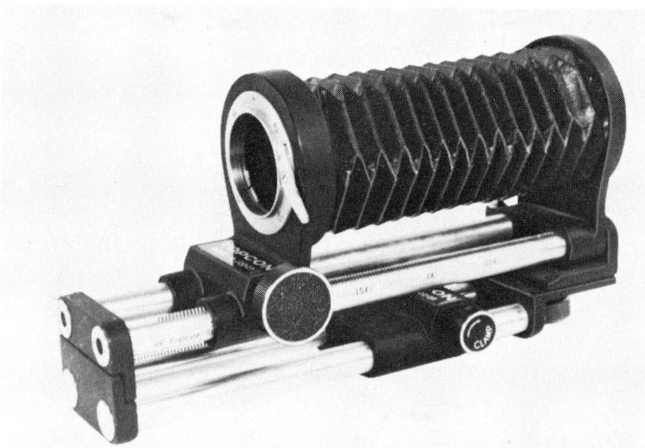

Fig. 7-6. The upper track of the bellows attachment provides variable magnification in close-up work; the lower track controls the focusing. (Courtesy of Beseler Topcon)

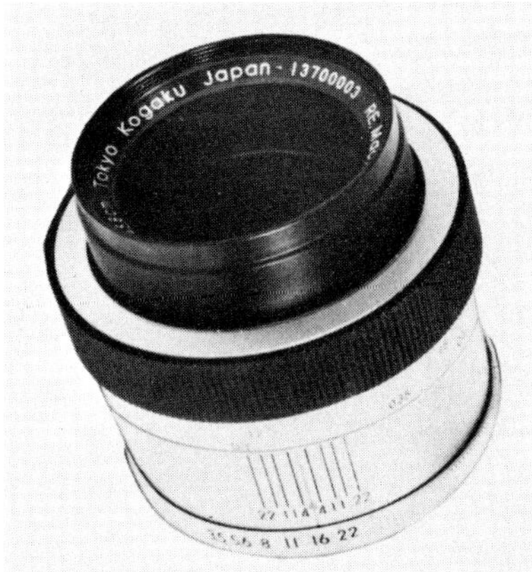

Fig. 7-7. Although designed specifically for close-up photograpy, the macro lens can also be focused out to infinity. However, because of its slow speed, it is generally not used in regular photography. (Courtesy of Beseler Topcon)

means of obtaining magnification in close-up photography. Available from +1 to +10 (above +10 would create too much distortion) and designed to fit over most normal lenses, the supplemental magnifying lens threads into the screw-type mount or can be inserted into a special adapter that fits the lens. Plus lenses do not give the same picture quality or variability of magnification that can be obtained by extending the lens from the camera.

Ring Light

When extension tubes, the bellows attachment or a macro lens is used for close-up dental photography, the distance between the camera and the orifice of the mouth being short, back or side lighting does not direct sufficient illumination into the oral cavity, and only a ring light can be employed as the light source. The ring light is an electronic flash designed to encircle the lens of the camera (Fig. 7-8). Since the light produced by a ring flash is shadowless and minimizes contrasts, pictures taken with it lack crispness. The resultant effect of using a ring light is acceptable for color work but poor for black-and-white photography.

Camera Set-ups

When choosing a camera arrangement for use in dental identification, the forensic dentist will be guided by the following considerations:

1. The amount of public, private or personal funds available to him for photographic equipment.

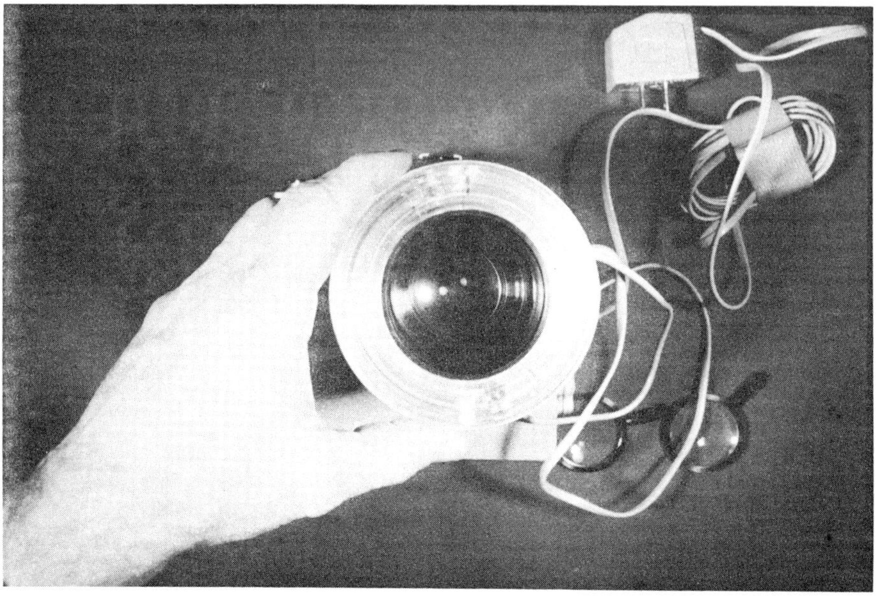

Fig. 7-8. The ring light is an electronic flash that encircles the lens of the camera, providing a shadowless light.

2. The extent of photographic knowledge that he has or plans to acquire.
3. The intended uses for his photographs.

Regarding the last, ordinarily photographs used in routine dental identification procedures are less critical than those intended for demonstrations, lectures and publications of various sorts. Ideally, the proposed utilization of the pictures would have the ultimate bearing on the photographic equipment selected. Although suggested primarily for use in dental identification, the photographic set-ups to be described here also can be used by law enforcement agencies for close-up evidence photography.

For quality pictures, a 35mm single-lens reflex camera (SLR) with through-the-lens metering (TTL) and interchangeable lenses should be used (see Fig. 7-4). Single-lens reflex means the viewing and focusing are both done by looking through the camera lens. By means of a mirror and prisms, the view through the lens is reflected in the eyepiece, and what is actually seen in the eyepiece will be recorded on the film. Such a system permits exact picture composition and precise focusing. Through-the-lens metering means the built-in light meter is behind the lens of the camera and measures the light coming

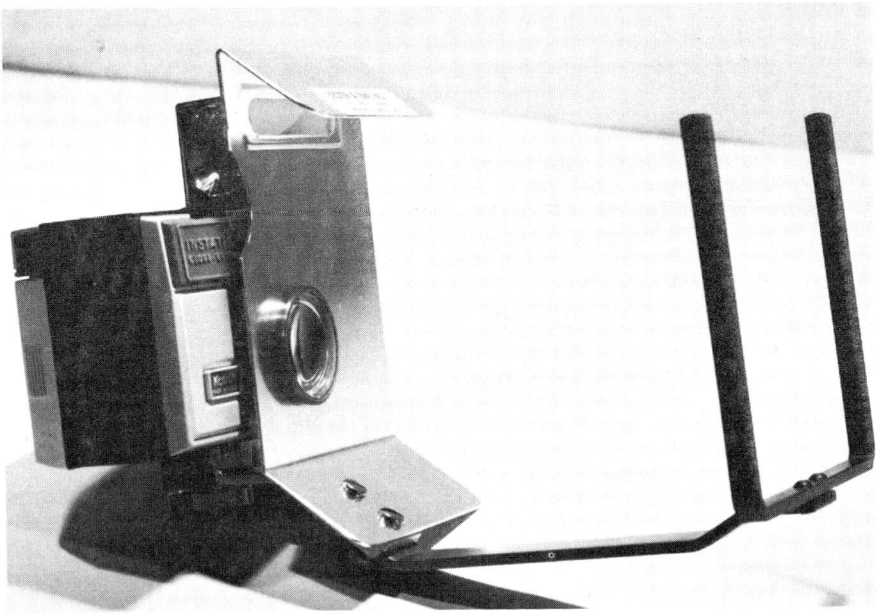

Fig. 7-9. The Kodak Instatech II close-up camera needs no adjustments for focus or aperture control. Matching the colored focal frame to the color-coded lens automatically puts the subject into proper focus within the frame. Light from the flashcube is controlled by a small, plastic window in the upper part of the lens frame.

through the lens opening. The meter pointer visible in the eyepiece indicates the proper aperture setting (*f*/stop) to be used.

There are many different camera arrangements suitable for close-up photography. Whichever is selected should be relatively simple to operate, inasmuch as during a routine postmortem examination the dentist does not have time to become involved in computing *f*/stops, varying exposure times or complex lighting components.

Three representative camera set-ups suitable for use in dental identification work are described below. Although any one of them will perform well and serve the needs of the forensic dentist, each exemplifies a different level in quality and professionalism of equipment, which will be reflected in the pictures produced.

Kodak Instatech II Close-up Camera

No previous photographic experience is necessary to operate the Kodak Instatech II close-up camera (Fig. 7-9), which has been de-

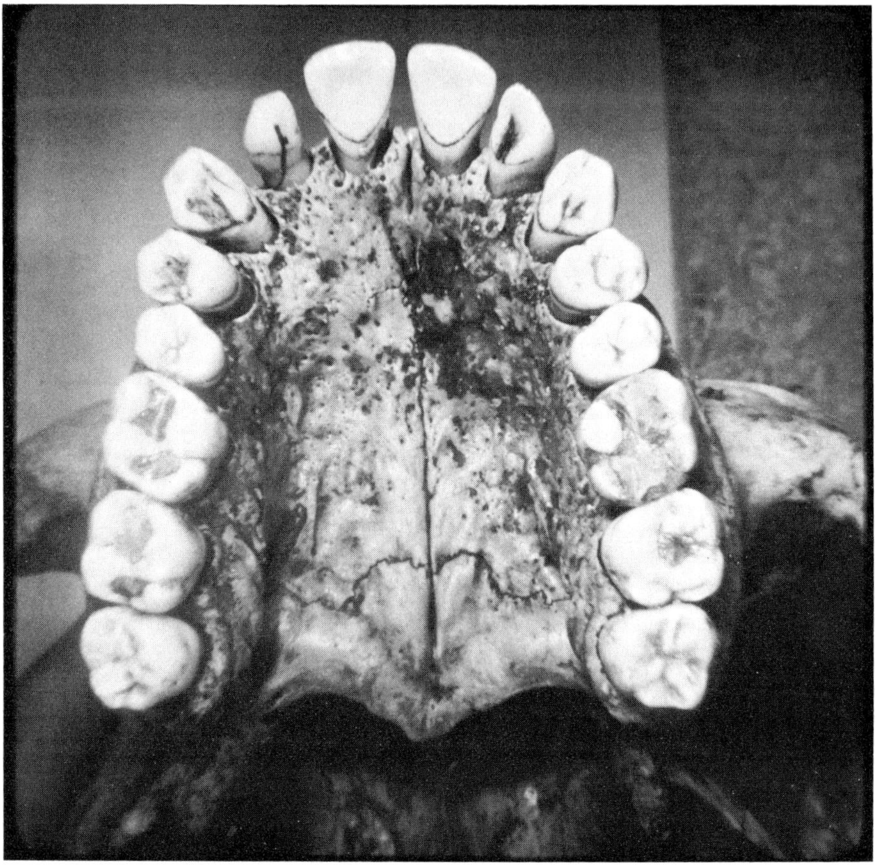

Fig. 7-10. Photograph taken with the Instatech II close-up camera, showing the square format.

signed specifically for close-up photography, embodying the principles of the Kodak Instamatic cameras. Easily loaded, the Instatech accepts all Kodak 126 cartridge films: Kodachrome-X or Ektachrome-X for color slides, Kodacolor-X for color prints and Verichrome Pan for black-and-white prints. Unlike 35mm film, which produces rectangular pictures, a 126 cartridge film produces a square format (Fig. 7-10). A flashcube is the light source for this set-up, enabling pictures to be taken indoors or outdoors regardless of lighting conditions.

Placing the color-coded lens and corresponding focal frame onto the camera automatically readies it for operation, providing the correct exposure with no settings to compute for distance and light,

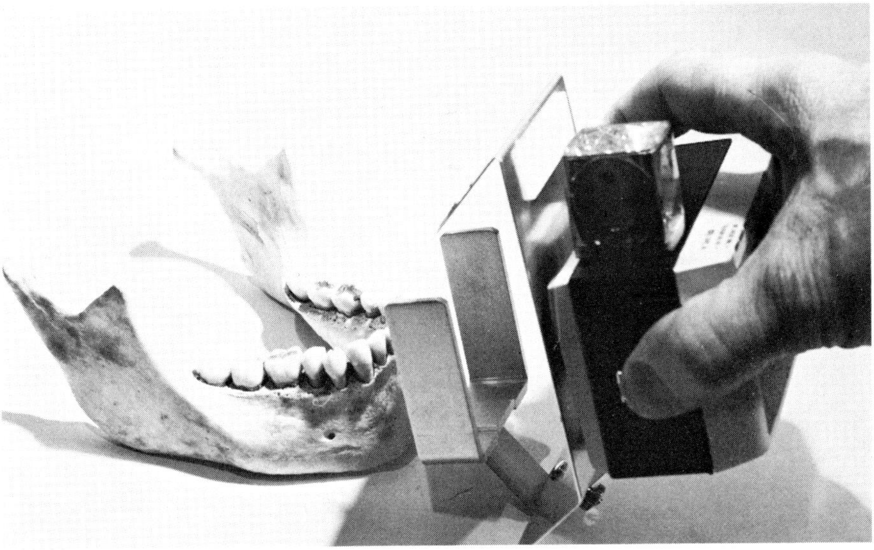

Fig. 7-11. At a distance of two inches from the subject, the Instatech II camera, equipped with the proper focal frame, is used to photograph a two-inch area.

or dials to adjust. Close-up photographs of small objects or of small areas of larger subjects are possible from a working distance of approximately 2 inches up to 24 inches and even to 36 inches, depending upon the lens, frame and film that are used (Fig. 7-11). The extremely small lens opening, *f*/32, results in great depth of field. (Depth of field refers to the zone of picture sharpness, which zone takes in the subject focused upon as well as objects in the foreground and background within a certain proximity to the subject. Generally, the smaller the aperture, or lens opening, the greater will be the depth of field.)

The basic Scientific Photo Outfit (approximately $56), includes the Kodak Instatech II close-up camera, two lenses and a frame.* The Deluxe Dental Kit (about $100) adds a carrying case and an additional lens attachment for close-ups at 2 inches from the subject. (Fig. 7-12).

Useful accessories include the data clip, a small holder for a strip of paper containing information to be photographed along with the subject so that the subject and information will appear together on one slide; a pair of double-end dental retractors, one side for children

* Lester A. Dine Inc., 2080 Jericho Turnpike, New Hyde Park, New York 11041

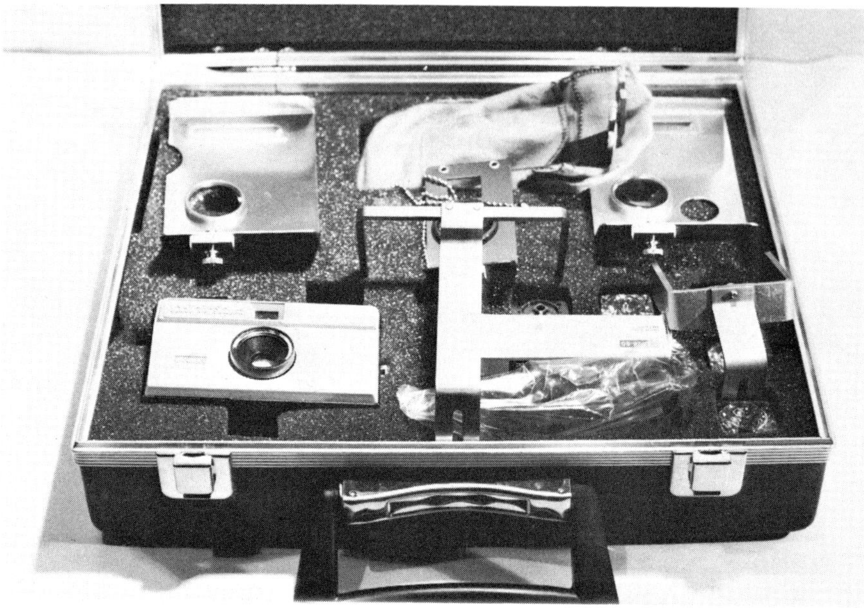

Fig. 7-12. The Deluxe Dental Kit, an inexpensive set-up for dental potography, includes the Instatech II camera, three lenses and a carrying case.

and the other for adults, and also for child or adult, polished metal, color-coded dental mouth mirrors, which fit directly on the camera for reflected pictures of the palate and occlusal surface of the teeth.

The Kodak Instatech II close-up camera is a simplified set-up particularly recommended for dentists and law enforcement officers with minimal knowledge of photography and for police departments with small budgets.

Dine Macro Lens Camera Set-up

The macro lens camera set-up for close-up photography utilizes a Minolta or Nikkormat 35mm SLR camera equipped with a macro lens, the Dine ring light and the Dine "quick focus programmer" (Fig. 7-13), a ring attachment that provides the correct aperture setting for the distance by means of a simple color scheme. Matching the color-coded *f*/stop to the color appearing on top of the rotating programmer attachment when the subject is in focus to the degree of magnification desired automatically sets the lens at the correct aperture for the exposure (Fig. 7-14). The Nikkormat FTN or Minolta

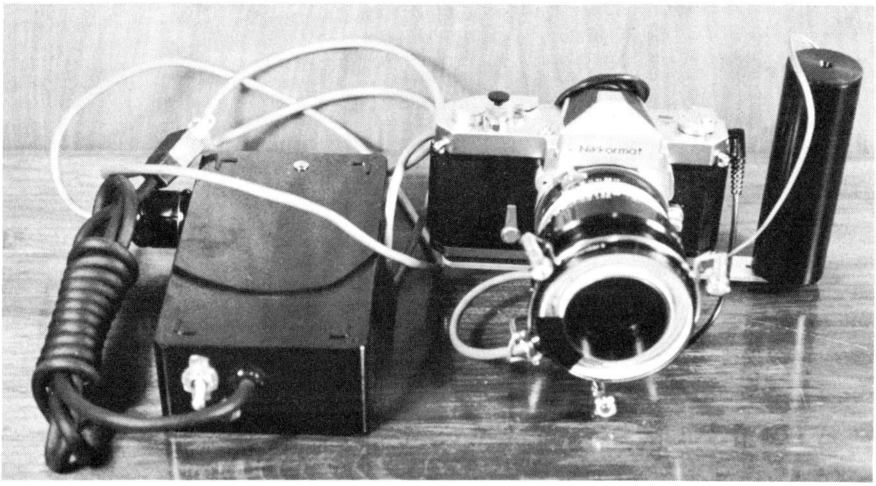

Fig. 7-13. The Nikkormat 35mm camera with the Nikon Micro lens, "quick focus programmer" and Dine ring light with power supply. This photographic set-up produces excellent color slides.

SRT-101 camera body with macro lens, quick programming ring and ring light with power supply is sold as a complete package (under $500).* Anyone already owning a Minolta or Nikkormat camera can purchase the components of the set-up separately.

Novoflex Automatic Diaphragm Lens and Bellows

The third camera rig for close-up photography combines the automatic Novoflex diaphragm lens and bellows with a quality 35mm SLR TTL camera (Fig. 7-15). This set-up comprises a four-track automatic bellows attachment, special short-mount Noflexar *f*/4 105mm lens with automatic diaphragm, a rotatable ring with shoe for electronic flash, and an anatomic pistol grip.

Depending on the make of the camera, the normal lens usually has a focal length of 45-58mm. The 105mm Noflexar lens is superior to the normal lens for close-up work for two reasons: (1) The normal lens, used with accessory devices, creates distortion in a three-dimensional subject image, whereas distortion is minimized by the long-focus lens (Fig. 7-16); (2) It allows greater working distance between the subject and lens, thus permitting better illumination of the subject.

* Lester A. Dine Inc., 2080 Jericho Turnpike, New Hyde Park, New York 11041.

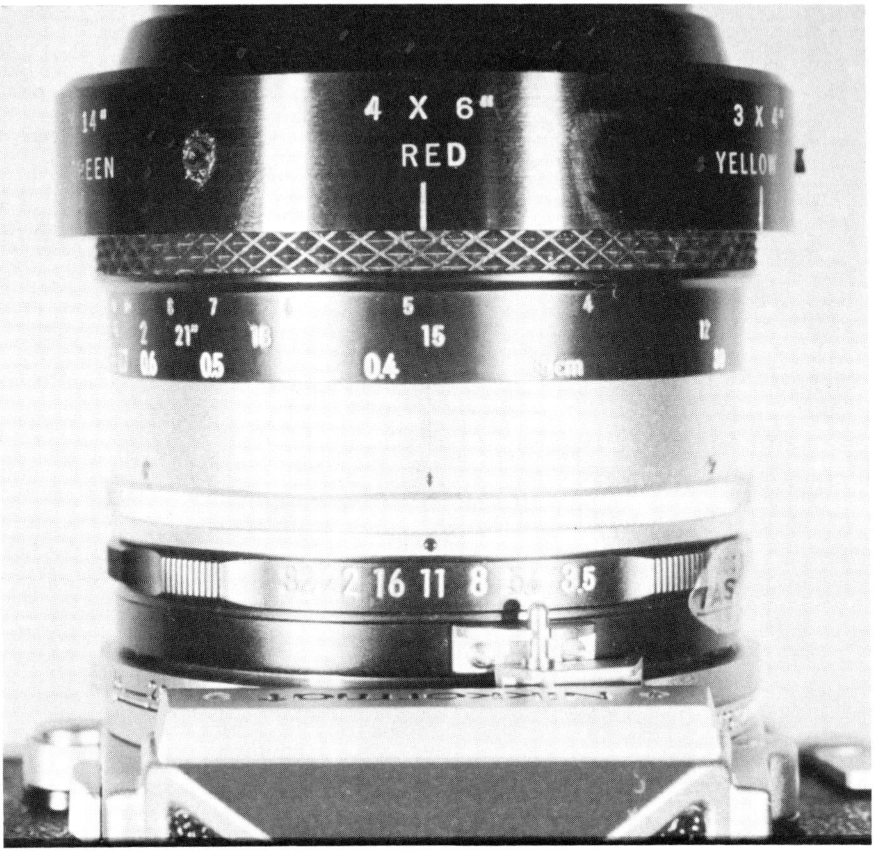

Fig. 7-14. The proper exposure is easily obtained with Dine's programmer attachment. Matching the color-coded *f*/stop to the color representing the desired degree of magnification automatically sets the lens at the correct aperture for the exposure.

The use of a short-mount long-focal-length lens with the bellows attachment enables focusing from infinity down to 1:1 (life-size). When on a regular mount connected to the bellows attachment, the long-focal-length lenses (90–105mm) do not focus to infinity.

A feature of most modern single-lens reflex cameras is the automatic diaphragm on the normal lens. The automatic diaphragm controls the size of the aperture, keeping the lens wide open during viewing and focusing. Coupled to the shutter mechanism, the automatic diaphragm, at the moment the shutter is released, closes down instantly to the preselected exposure setting and then returns auto-

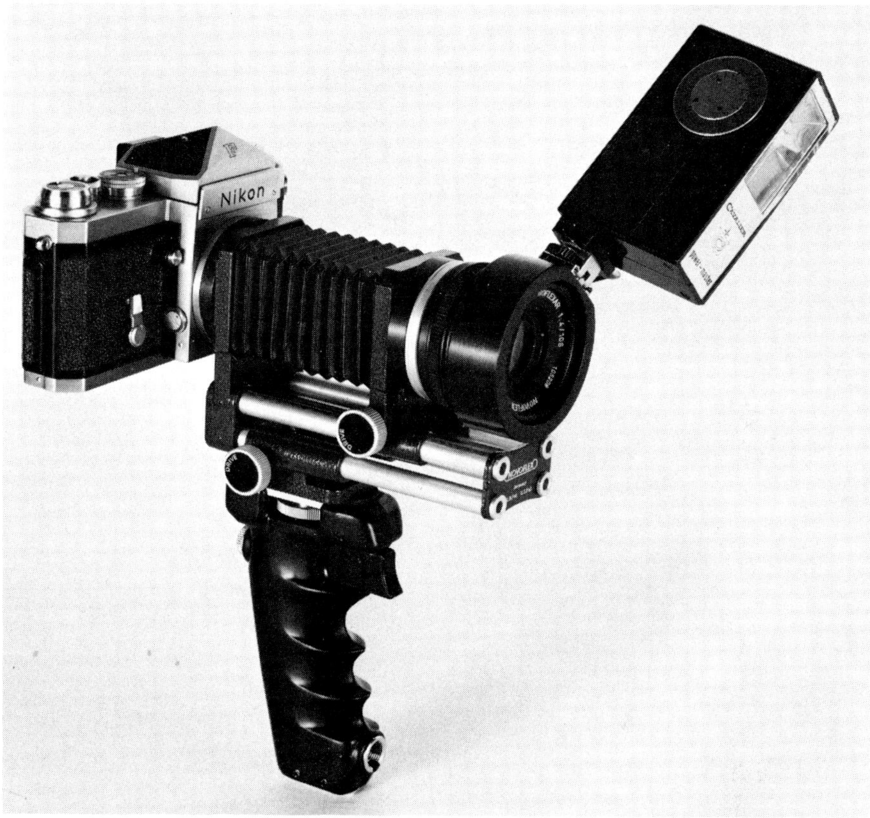

Fig. 7-15. A 35mm camera equipped with the Novoflex bellows attachment and short mount auto-diaphragm lens permits photographs to be taken from infinity down to life size at 1 : 1. (Courtesy of Burleigh Brooks Optics, Inc.)

matically to its fully open state. The diaphragm does not operate automatically, however, when the normal lens is affixed to the ordinary bellows attachment for close-up work.

Without the automatic bellows, the aperture must be closed down to the correct *f*/stop prior to exposure, darkening the viewing screen so that focusing is extremely difficult. To remedy that deficiency, present with an ordinary bellows attachment, a double cable release (Fig. 7-17) can be connected to the lens and camera. Using the cable to control the diaphragm manually makes it possible to keep the aperture fully open until just before the shutter is released.

The Novoflex arrangement for close-up photography features the

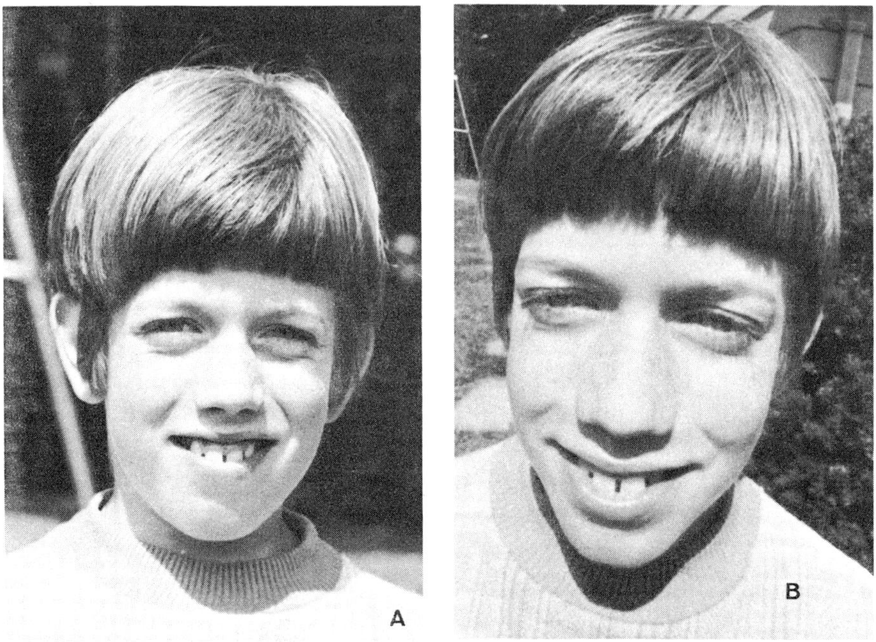

Fig. 7-16. When a three-dimensional object is photographed too close to the camera lens, optical distortion is produced. *A*, Photograph taken with 100mm lens at a distance of five feet from the subject. *B*, Photograph taken with 20mm lens at a distance of one foot from the subject exaggerates the distortion that occurs when a subject, although in focus, is photographed too close to the camera lens.

automatic diaphragm long-focus lens coupled to a 35mm SLR camera through the automatic bellows attachment. The Novoflex automatic bellows, which fits most 35mm cameras, including Nikon, Nikkormat, Pentax, Minolta and Topcon, permits viewing and focusing at full aperture when used with the normal camera lens or the Noflexar 4.0/105mm long-focus lens.

Lighting for this set-up is provided by any small electronic flash having an accurate guide number of 40 with Kodachrome II film (ASA 25). A friction-fit, rotatable ring with shoe holds the strobe (electronic flash) on the lens. The ring pushes on to a rubber knurl on the auto-Noflexar lens and rotates to give the best light modeling. The location of the point light source (strobe) is based on the inverse square law: When the bellows is extended for greater magnification, additional light is required. The strobe, mounted to the lens, moves

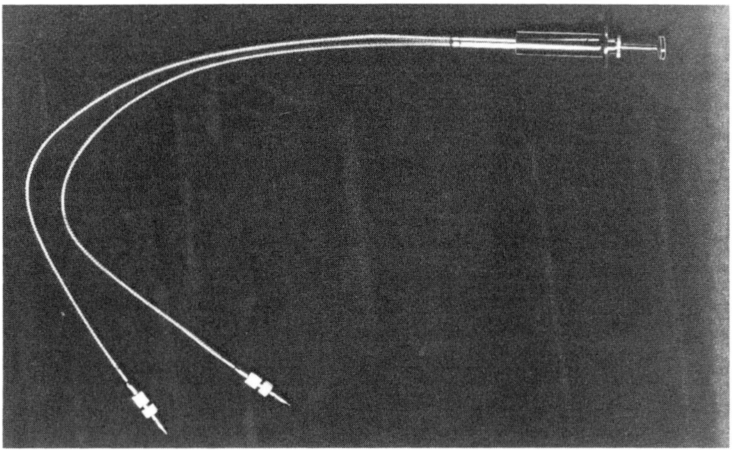

Fig. 7-17. A double cable release provides individual, manual control of the diaphragm and the shutter mechanism. (Courtesy of Beseler Topcon)

backward and forward with the lens, spontaneously increasing the illumination as the lens moves toward the subject and decreasing the illumination as the lens moves away from the subject.

Once the exposure has been determined, it remains constant, eliminating any further calculations. A constant aperture of *f*/22 will usually suffice for all lens-to-subject distances from $2\frac{1}{2}$ feet to 8 inches (1:1). The aperture setting for pictures taken at a distance greater than $2\frac{1}{2}$ feet can be determined by dividing the film guide number of the strobe (40) by the distance (e.g., at $3\frac{1}{2}$ feet the aperture would be *f*/11).

The Novoflex automatic bellows and long-focus lens kit,* ($199.50 excluding camera and flash) is available through local camera dealers.

* Burleigh Brooks Optics, Inc., 44 Burlews Court, Hackensack, New Jersey 07601.

8 Antemortem Records

A dental identification becomes necessary with the recovery of a deceased unable to be identified by other means. The discovery of a body is indicative of a missing person, whether reported missing or not. Since some sort of comparative antemortem record is essential in order to make a dental identification of a body, information of a missing person is generally a prerequisite for obtaining antemortem dental records. If no missing person has been reported who might relate to the body, then in all probability, no dental comparison will be possible.

The science of dental identification is based on the astronomical number of different combinations possible in the dental charting of the human mouth. Moreover, because the teeth and restorations are highly resistant to destruction after death, it is likely that they will be recovered postmortem. In the process of establishing a dental identification (DID) there are four major steps: (1) examining the oral region, (2) preparing postmortem records, (3) securing antemortem records, (4) comparing antemortem with postmortem records.

Following completion of the postmortem examination and associative procedures, the forensic dentist will procure antemortem records, if they were not obtained earlier. The search for dental records of a missing person lies within the jurisdiction of the forensic dentist, inasmuch as he is continuing the chain of evidence that he initiated in the case. At times, more hours are spent in sleuthing than were required to examine, chart, x-ray and photograph the body. Although, in general, the police are unfamiliar with what can constitute dental evidence and how to acquire it, a good investigating officer, working under the direction of the dentist can save him time and effort.

Commonly, a dental identification is based on a comparison of the antemortem dental chart and x-rays with the postmortem dental chart and x-rays. Questionable aspects, however, may diminish or nullify the usefulness of the antemortem record. If the victim's antemortem dental records were prepared many years before death, the forensic dentist, aware that the older the record the more likely there are to be inconsistencies due to changes in the mouth, must be satisfied that any discrepancies are attributable to the time lapse. If that does not account for them, then either the value of the particular antemortem evidence is suspect or the victim is not the missing person.

A wide variance exists in the quality of antemortem charting. Many dental records are detailed, accurate and professionally executed, whereas some are surprisingly slipshod, with scanty details and gross inaccuracies. Dental identification having emerged as a valid, viable science, more than ever it is incumbent upon every dentist to maintain good dental records and to retain them for a substantial period—at least ten years.

COMMON ANTEMORTEM RECORDS

Dental Charts

There is a plethora of different kinds of antemortem dental record cards. Most combine some form of diagrammatic chart of the dentition with a verbal description of the treatment rendered (Fig. 8-1). The anatomical diagrammatic drawing is preferable to the nonanatomical (Fig. 8-2) because it is easier on the anatomic drawing to delineate the shapes and sizes of restorations. Dentists who utilize verbal charting entirely use a record card without a diagrammatic chart, preferring to write out a detailed account of the treatment they have rendered the patient. The antemortem diagrammatic representation of the dentition is more readily compared with the postmortem chart, a consideration of particular importance in a mass disaster.

Typical information contained in the record card includes the dates of treatments, teeth treated, surfaces restored and restorative materials used. The construction of a partial or full denture is noted, usually along with the shade of tooth selected. Omitted, for the most part, are the mold numbers, type of posterior teeth and the partial denture design. In crown and bridgework, generally the number of units is recorded and, occasionally, the type of abutments that were used. Although the dentist often marks carious lesions and missing

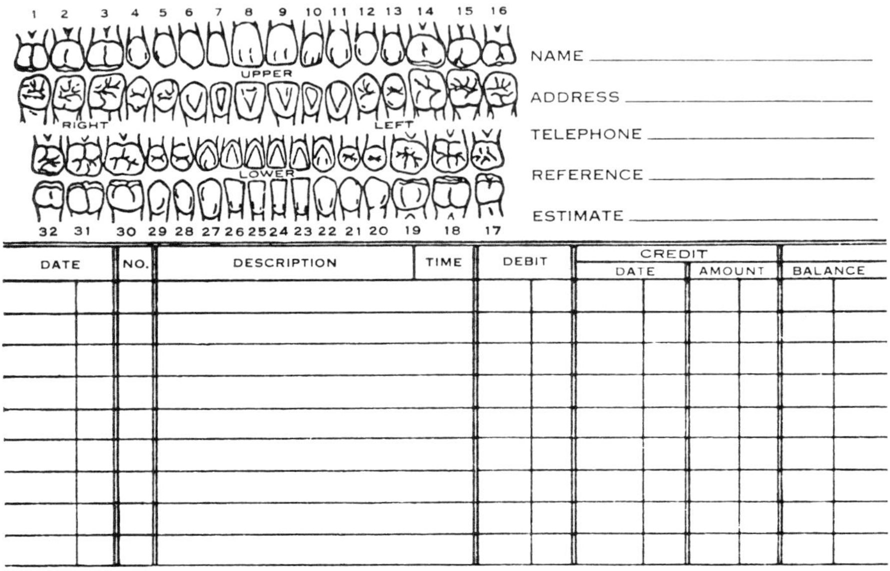

Fig. 8-1. Typical dental record card used in the United States, containing anatomical diagrammatic chart and space for a verbal description of the professional services rendered. There are many hundreds of different dental record cards currently in use.

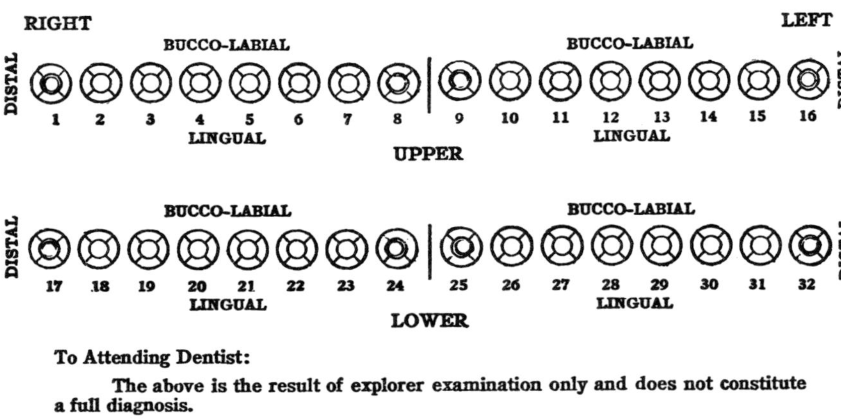

Fig. 8-2. A nonanatomical diagrammatic chart used in the employee dental clinic of The Travelers Insurance Companies in Hartford. System of dental notation is similar to that formerly used by the U.S. Navy.

teeth on the diagrammatic chart, seldom does he take the time to mark those teeth that were restored prior to his own treatment procedures.

Dental X-rays

For comparative purposes in dental identification, the x-ray, owing to its dependable, precise reproduction of details, is the most desirable antemortem record. Unfortunately, many dentists dispose of their patients' x-rays after a year or two. The most likely sources for antemortem dental x-rays, besides the general dentist, are dental specialists, such as the orthodontist, endodontist, periodontist and oral surgeon; the Armed Services, and various institutions, such as a dental clinic, hospital, prison, mental health center, etc.

The kinds of x-rays used in dentistry are bite-wing, periapical, occlusal, panoramic and lateral plate. The first three are classified as intra-oral because the film is held within the mouth during exposure. The panoramic and lateral plate films, classified as extra-oral, are external to the mouth during exposure. Each type of x-ray film is used to obtain a specific view of the dentition and comes in a standard size that, nonetheless, may vary slightly from one manufacturer to another.

Bite-wing. The interproximal x-ray is commonly referred to as the bite-wing because, in order to hold the film in position during exposure, the patient grips a wing tab between the upper and lower teeth on the side of the mouth. The bite-wing reveals the supporting bone crests, caries on the proximal surfaces of the coronal and cervical regions of the teeth, the internal configuration of restorations and the cement bases under them. Since a single film shows the posterior teeth on one side of the mouth of both the maxilla and mandible, only two x-rays are needed for a representative view of both sides of the mouth, making the bite-wing particularly suited for use as antemortem evidence in dental identification. The approximate size of No. 3 posterior bite-wing film is $2\frac{1}{2} \times 1\frac{1}{16}$ inches.

Periapical. The periapical x-ray reproduces the entire tooth and its surrounding structures. The standard periapical measures, approximately, $1\frac{1}{4} \times 1\frac{5}{8}$ inches and normally includes up to three teeth on a film.

Occlusal. Used to detect root fragments, unerupted teeth and pathological conditions in large areas of the maxilla and mandible, occlusal

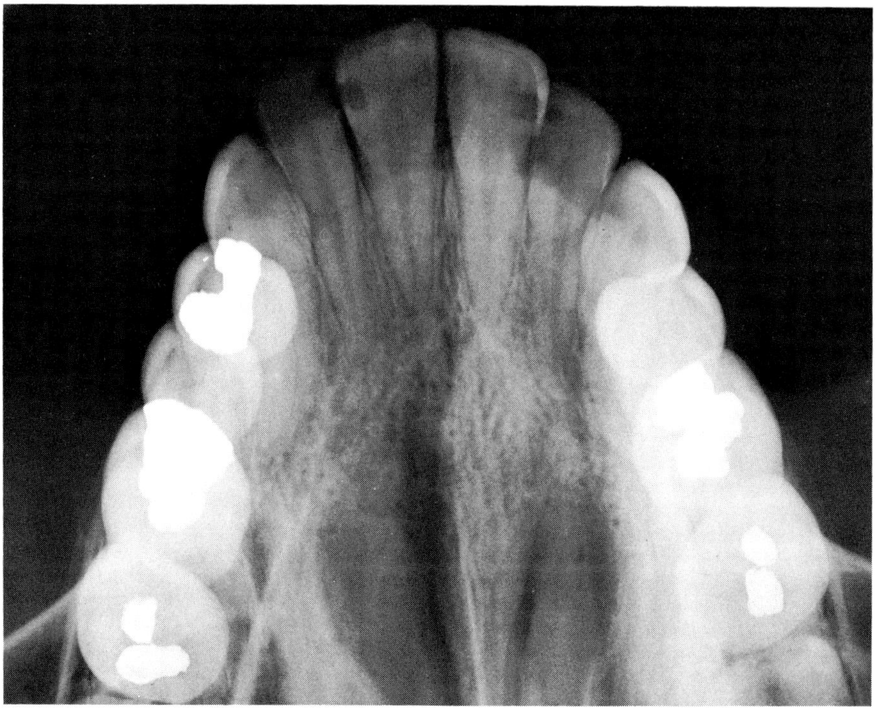

Fig. 8-3. Because it is seldom included in antemortem dental records, the occlusal x-ray is rarely used postmortem.

film (Fig. 8-3) is so called because it is placed on the occlusal plane for exposure. The approximate size is $2\frac{1}{4} \times 3$ inches.

Panoramic. The United States Army recently discontinued the use of written dental charts for identification and substituted, instead, the antemortem panoramic x-ray of the dentition. A single film, approximately 5×12 inches, encompasses a complete view of the dentition, showing both the mandibular and maxillary anterior and posterior teeth and the surrounding structures. Because the entire dentition is reproduced in one antemortem film that can be easily scanned, the panoramic roentgenogram is ideal for use in dental identification, especially in a mass disaster. Manufacturers of panoramic x-ray equipment include General Electric, S. S. White (Fig. 8-4) and Siemens.

Lateral Plate. Used in dentistry mainly by orthodontists and oral surgeons to x-ray large areas of the dentition from outside the

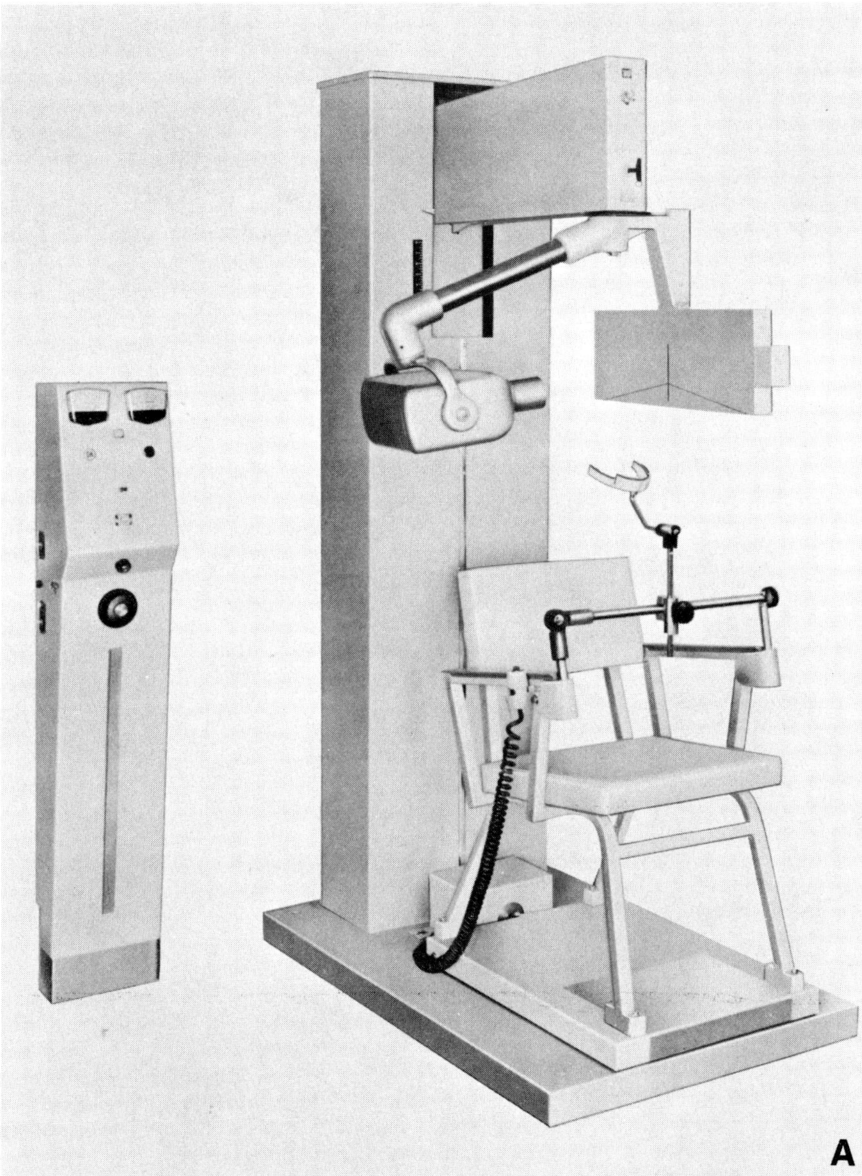

Fig. 8-4. A, Panorex machine made by S. S. White takes panoramic x-rays. (Courtesy of S. S. White Company)

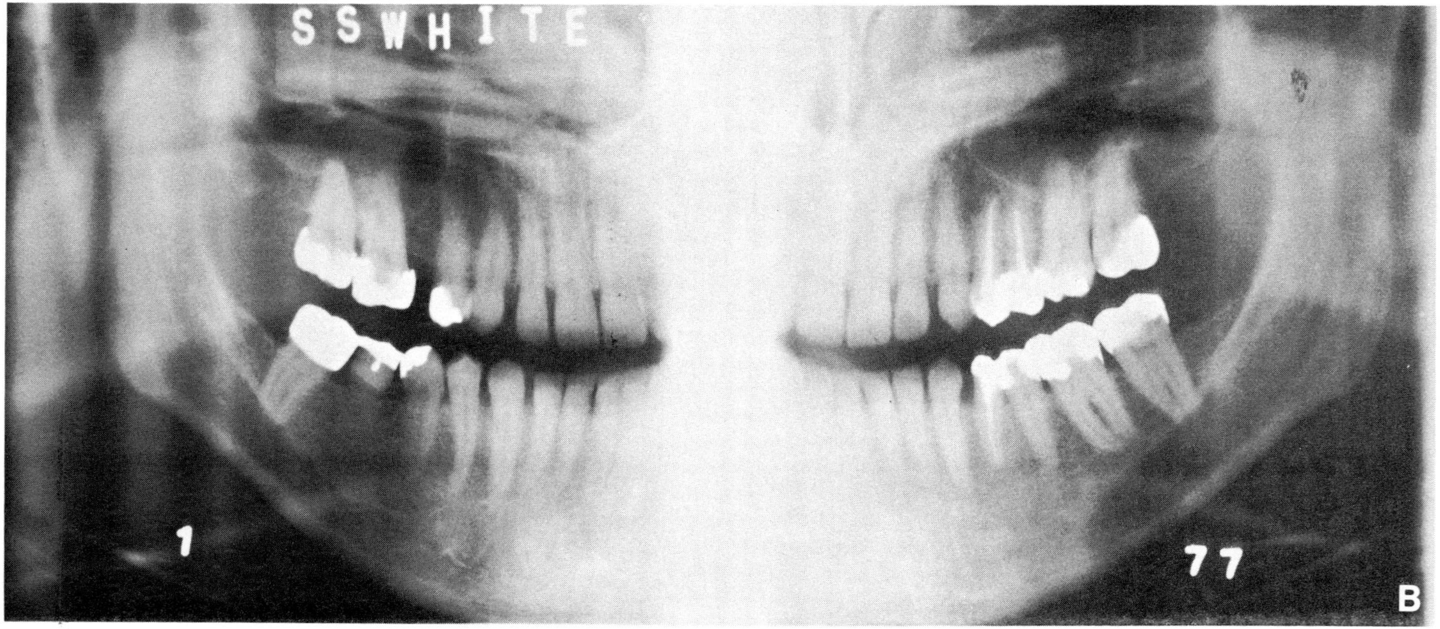

Fig. 8-4. B, Since a single film shows the entire dentition, the panoramic x-ray is an excellent antemortem record for use in dental identification.

mouth, the lateral plate radiograph, 8 × 10 inches, is, generally, unsatisfactory for use in dental identification because it often shows the teeth and restorations in superimposition, obscuring details (Fig. 8-5). It is the x-ray easiest to take postmortem.

ADDITIONAL ANTEMORTEM EVIDENCE

The common antemortem dental records, that is, x-rays and diagrammatic and verbal charting, are not the only means to a valid dental identification. When the more familiar antemortem dental records are unobtainable or, for one reason or another, are unsatisfactory, then the forensic dentist is forced to go farther afield in his search for acceptable antemortem evidence that can be used in establishing an identification. Because each case is individual, the dentist is required, at times, to be innovative not only in his handling of the postmortem procedures but also in searching for antemortem information. Other evidence that could contribute to establishing a dental identification includes study models, prosthetic appliances, medical records and x-rays, photographs and—under particular circumstances—sworn statements.

Study Models

Orthodontists make extensive use of study models for case planning and the constructing of orthodontic appliances. Moreover, these models are generally retained over an extended period of time. Only occasionally does the general dentist make study models of the patient before commencing a program of treatment, and rarely does he retain them for long. Although orthodontic study models are not commonly used as antemortem evidence, in the situation where dental charts and x-rays are unavailable and the orthodontic models are the only antemortem record, they can be the basis for a dental identification.

Case History

A body decomposed beyond recognition was recovered from the West River in New Haven, Connecticut, and removed to the morgue at Yale-New Haven Hospital. As an accommodation, the jaws were resected by the hospital pathologist and brought by police car to the forensic dentist in Hartford. At the time of the postmortem dental examination, the only antemortem dental record available was a set

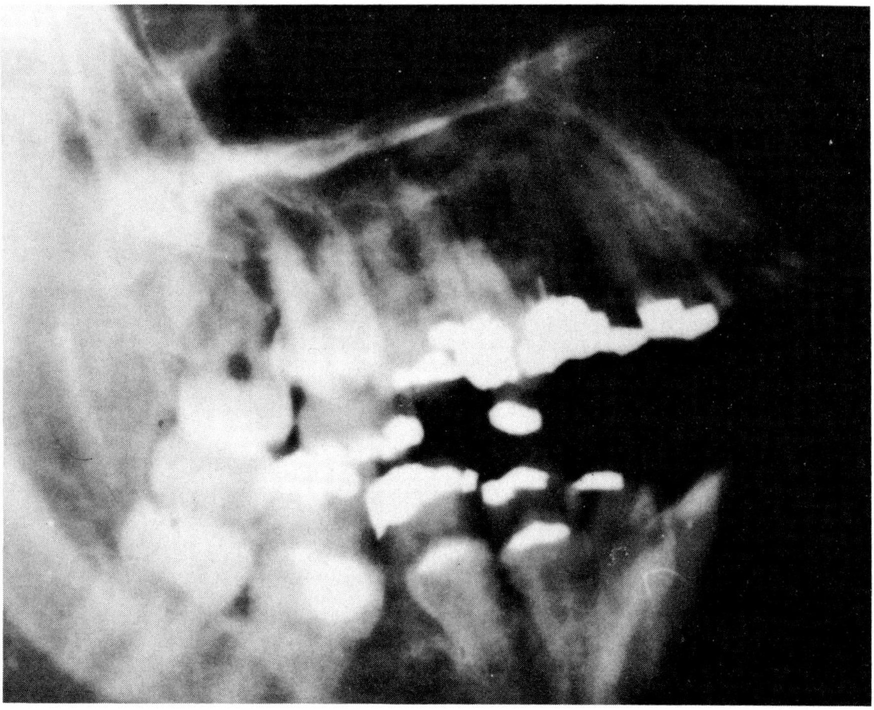

Fig. 8-5. In the lateral plate x-ray, the teeth and restorations often appear superimposed and indistinct, making it the least suitable type of x-ray for use in dental identification.

of orthodontic study models that had been made ten years earlier. Comparing the jaws with the models enabled an immediate identification to be made (Fig. 8-6). Later, corroborative antemortem x-rays were obtained from the victim's general dentist.

Prosthetic Appliances

Bridgework and dentures in the mouth of an unidentified deceased may yield much information for comparison with antemortem dental evidence. When another denture belonging to a person presumed to be the deceased is available for use as antemortem evidence, it is possible for an identification to be based on comparable aspects in both appliances. The rugae, being immutable and individual, are a superior and infallible criterion for comparing dentures. Other comparable characteristics may show a degree of variation incident to changes in the mouth, especially if a long time has elapsed between the construction of the two dentures. The following case is

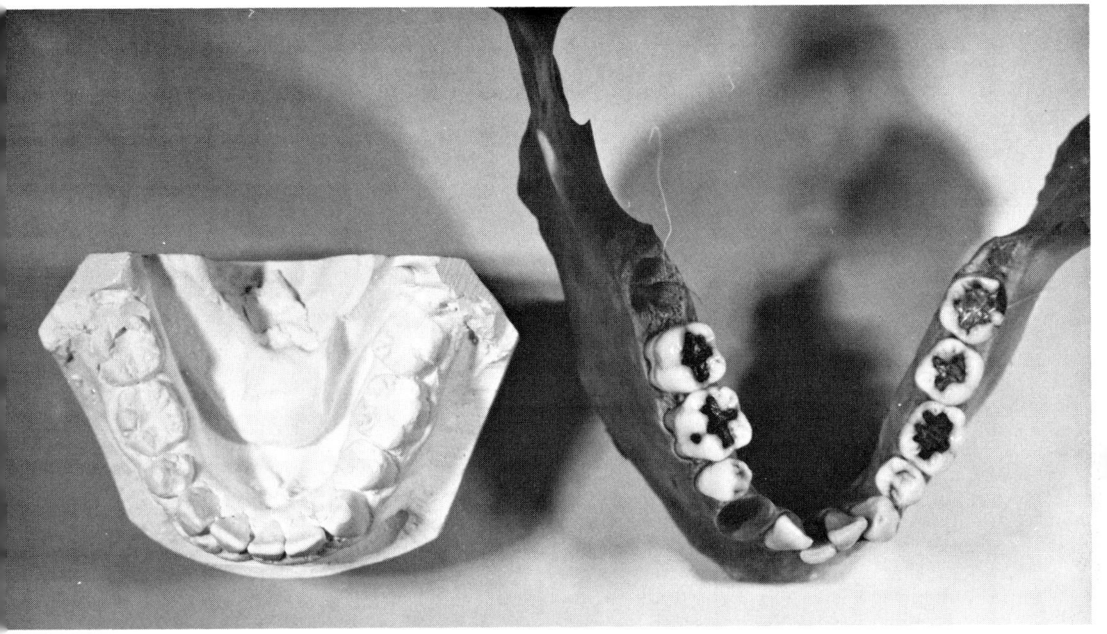

Fig. 8-6. Resected mandible next to orthodontic mandibular model of victim. Identification was based on a comparison of the dentition with the orthodontic models made ten years before.

unique in that a dental identification was made through a single prosthetic appliance.

Case History

A car sideswiped in downtown Hartford flipped over and was quickly engulfed in flames. The driver and sole occupant, entrapped when his foot was caught under the brake pedal, was burned beyond recognition. The police had the body removed to a nearby funeral home.

It was learned from the family of the victim, who had been tentatively identified through the license plates on the car, that he had last been to a dentist fifteen years before to have an abcessed lower molar extracted. The molar had been an abutment tooth for a four-unit fixed bridge that was removed at the time of the extraction. The dentist had records for the rest of the family but not of the victim.

Meanwhile, the son recalled that his father, rather than discarding the bridge, had retained it in a bureau drawer to sell, eventually,

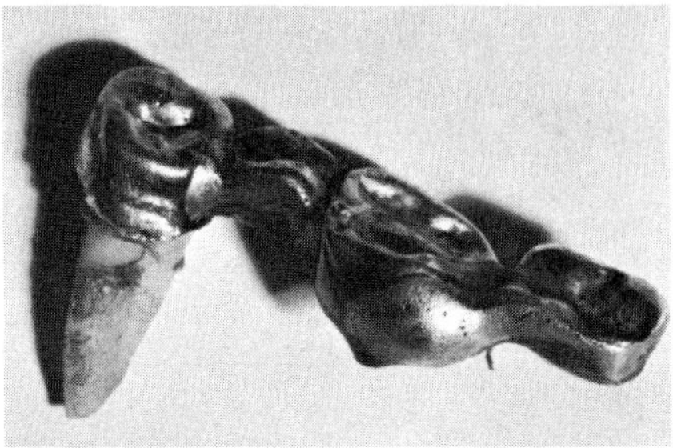

Fig. 8-7. Since there were no other dental records, the victim's fixed bridge, removed 15 years before death, was the basis for identification. It fitted perfectly on bicuspid tooth, shown here extracted postmortem.

for the scrap gold value. Inserted into the mouth of the deceased, the bridge matched the space in the dentition and fitted perfectly onto the remaining abutment tooth, a lower bicuspid. Thus, without benefit of written records, identity was confirmed by a prosthetic appliance that had been out of the mouth for fifteen years (Fig. 8-7).

Medical Records and X-rays

Included with a patient's medical history may be a brief, general description of his dentition as observed by the examining physician. Although the verbal charting may contain some inconsequential inaccuracies attributable to the physician's limited knowledge of dentistry, it may still provide enough essential data on which to base a dental identification.

Since medical x-rays of the head and neck frequently show the dentition, they may prove useful for identification. As an example of this, a chiropractor's lateral plate skull and neck x-rays, clearly revealing the dentition of a victim burned to death in an automobile accident, constituted acceptable antemortem evidence for the dental identification when no dental records were available.

Photographs

Dental. Occasionally a dentist may take oral photographs of a patient before commencing treatment and again upon concluding treatment. Such close-up views of the dentition may, in some instances, constitute a satisfactory antemortem record for use in identification, especially where unusual dental characteristics are evident.

Nondental. In the nondental photograph taken by an amateur or professional photographer, the subject often smiles broadly, exposing a large area of the dentition. Studying the picture under a strong magnifying glass or scrutinizing an enlargement, if the picture was taken with good photographic equipment, may enable detection of missing, discolored, broken or chipped teeth, a malocclusion or other

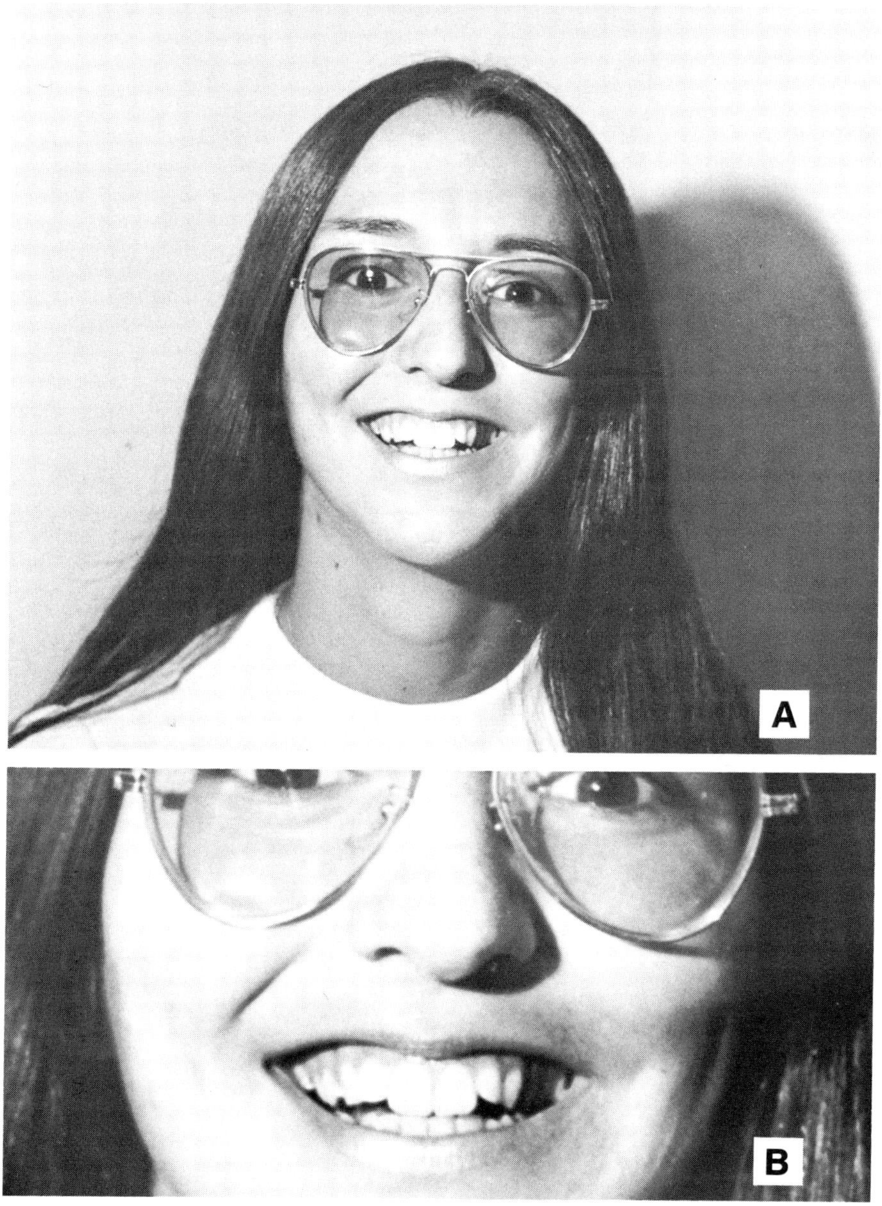

Fig. 8-8. A, Nondental photograph of smiling subject reveals broad area of dentition. *B,* Photographic enlargement of the dentition discloses a malocclusion, which might be a clue to identification.

dental conditions (Fig. 8-8). Though it is doubtful that a nondental photograph would be the sole basis for an identification, it is, nonetheless, possible for it to be the determinant of an exclusion, especially if it clearly exhibits antemortem details not evident in the dentition of the deceased.

Sworn Statements

When all efforts to obtain some sort of concrete antemortem record have failed, the forensic dentist is forced to resort to less orthodox evidence in a final attempt to arrive at an identification. In an exceptional case the carefully taken testimony of lay persons might be used in dental identification.

Case History

A fire occurred in a third-rate rooming house in Waterbury, Connecticut, burning to death eight of the residents. Of the five burned beyond recognition, four were identified through dental records. The last unidentified body, presumed to be the missing person, was an alcoholic with, according to the family, no record of dental treatment. The victim was edentulous in the maxilla and was missing a lower front tooth.

The forensic dentist directed the assisting police officer to locate persons who knew the missing man and could furnish a description of his dentition. The detective was cautioned against inadvertently disclosing suggestive information to anyone undergoing questioning.

Four friends of the missing person were found, each one affirming separately that the deceased had no upper teeth and was missing a lower front tooth. The detective also located a former girlfriend who claimed to have been with the victim the night he used a pair of pliers to extract his lower front tooth. Sworn statements were made by all five.

In addition, an alcoholic clinic where the victim had once been a patient furnished medical reports for 1967 and 1969, which stated that at the time of treatment he was edentulous in the maxilla. Dental identification was based on the depositions and the two medical reports. Other professional opinions concurred on acceptance of the attestations as evidence, under the circumstances.

SEEKING ANTEMORTEM INFORMATION

Conversational Clues

When antemortem dental records of a body have not yet been obtained, friends or relatives of the victim may be able to furnish the name of a dentist who treated the deceased. Failing that, they may be able to describe specific dental characteristics in the victim, such as missing or discolored teeth, gold crowns, a protruding jaw, or other dental details that may contribute to an eventual identification. Conversational information, while not in itself the basis for an identification, may lead, directly or indirectly, to the acquisition of acceptable antemortem evidence and a resultant identification.

Occupational and Oral Correlations

The occupation or avocation of the deceased may bear a correlation to certain characteristics possibly present in the dentition, for example:

threadbiting seamstress—notched teeth
chemical factory employee—chemical deposits on the teeth and in gum tissue
candy factory employee—excessive caries from sugar dust
musician (reed instruments)—malocclusion produced by mouthpiece.

Wanted–Information Bulletin

A request for information inserted in the newspapers, possibly accompanied by a suitable picture of the deceased, or a Wanted—Information bulletin published in a dental journal along with a photograph, postmortem dental chart or the prints of x-rays might yield either the desired antemortem evidence or leads for follow-up.

Case History

The custodian of a large apartment house in Hartford, Connecticut, complained to the police about a foul odor emanating from a third floor apartment rented to a 36-year-old assistant college professor. The occupant, who had a history of mental illness, had not been seen in over three weeks.

On entering the apartment, the police found on the bed a badly decomposed body covered with maggots. Nearby was an open bottle of barbiturates. The victim's father, notified in West Virginia, planned to fly to Hartford the next day with another son to claim the body. Since neither visual nor fingerprint identification was possible, a forensic dentist was called into the case with the hope that a dental identification could be made before the family's arrival.

Following the postmortem dental procedures, the search for antemortem dental records was begun. Neither the family nor friends of the deceased were able to furnish the name of a dentist to whom the victim might have gone. As a last resort, a news item was published in a metropolitan newspaper, requesting any dentist who had treated the professor to make contact with the Hartford Police Department. The next morning, the professor's dentist from New Britain saw the article and telephoned the police. Within an hour the antemortem dental records were delivered to the forensic dentist, enabling an identification to be made shortly before the arrival of the victim's family.

Police Inquiry

The forensic dentist should guide the assisting police officer in the attempt to discover the whereabouts of antemortem dental records. Following are a few suggested leads that might be pursued in the quest for antemortem information:

1. When questioning the family of a missing person who may be the deceased, ask for the names and addresses of dentists who have treated the missing person.

2. Did the missing person have dental insurance or belong to a union dental plan? Did he ever go for treatment to a medical or dental clinic?

3. If he was in the military reserves or was a service veteran, obtain information on the branch of service, rank, serial number, social security number and dates of active duty. The Armed Services or Veterans Administration may have antemortem dental records.

4. If a criminal record is found, ascertain whether the deceased ever served time in a correctional institution, and if so, where and when? A prison may have antemortem dental records.

5. Was the missing person ever confined to a mental hospital or a retention center for alcoholics or drug addicts? If dental care was rendered, dental records may be available. The rampant caries often seen in the mouth of the drug addict may be a clue to identification.

Once given the names of dentists who treated the missing person, the forensic dentist should make the initial contact himself, usually a telephone call explaining the situation and requesting antemortem dental records. A personal relationship is both conducive to cooperation and less inhibiting to the dentist being questioned, allowing him to converse freely using the professional terminology to which he is accustomed. If dental charts are available, the odontologist should ask the system used for designating the teeth and whether the record cards contain code symbols that need interpreting.

TRANSMITTING DENTAL DATA

When the antemortem dental records have been located, their mode of conveyance to the forensic dentist will be contingent upon the urgency, distance and facilities available. To reduce the chance of loss in transit, records should be carefully packaged. Dental x-rays especially, because they are usually small, can easily slip out of envelopes left unsealed or unstapled.

If the return of the original antemortem records has been requested, the x-rays can be duplicated (see Chapter 6) and the written records should be reproduced by a copying machine. The duplicate records remain with the file on the deceased; the original records should be returned by first-class mail.

Police Conveyance

Police conveyance, which can be done in relays if the distance is great or interstate boundaries are crossed, is a fast, reliable way of transporting dental records from the source to the forensic odontologist. At each transferral point a signed receipt should be obtained, thereby maintaining a continuous chain should it become necessary to trace back for any reason (see Fig. 2-3).

Telephone Transmission

Verbal transmission of the antemortem records over the telephone is resorted to only when the circumstances of the case demand an immediate identification of the deceased and do not allow sufficient time for forwarding the written records. A tape recording of the telephone conversation, made with the telephone pick-up accessory (see Fig. 3-11*B*), is a valuable adjunct. Having first ascertained from the dentist the system of tooth designation used, the forensic odontologist, transcribing all the information, should request a complete reading of the dental chart and x-rays, including a description, with dates, of dental services rendered. Even though the telephone conversation enables an identification to be made, the antemortem records should still be sent to the forensic dentist as verification.

U.S. Postal Service

First-Class. A relatively safe way of transporting dental records, first-class mail is the fastest mail service for short distances; for long distances airmail should be used. Even when closed to other types of mail, the post office usually has a place allocated for the receipt, at any time, of outgoing first-class mail. And, of course, it can always be placed in an outdoor mailbox.

Certified. Certified mail provides the same service as first-class with, additionally, a record of delivery. For a return receipt of delivery, there is an extra fee.

Registered. Often slower than first-class mail because signatures are required of all handlers, registered mail, since it is the safest type of postal service, is recommended for x-rays and other valuable records. At the time of registration, which can be done only when the post office window is open, a record of mailing is issued. Like certified mail, there is also a record of delivery and an added charge for a return receipt of delivery. The records of accountable mail, certified and registered, are retained by the post office for two years.

Special Delivery. Added to other mail service, special delivery provides for prompt delivery from the destination post office to the addressee. Probably the most suitable mail service for dental records going beyond 150 miles would be first-class registered airmail with special delivery added. The approximate costs for this are 11 cents—Airmail, per ounce, 95 cents—Registered, 60 cents—Special Delivery.

Facsimile Transmission Equipment

The Xerox Telecopier delivers fast, accurate reproductions of all kinds of written matter—printed, penned, penciled, typewritten. Even the diagrammatic dental chart is easily transmitted by Telecopier. Compact, lightweight and portable, the unit can be set up wherever there is a conventional telephone and a 110V electrical outlet. Although the telephone lines are used for transmission, no direct connection to the telephone is required (Fig. 8-9).

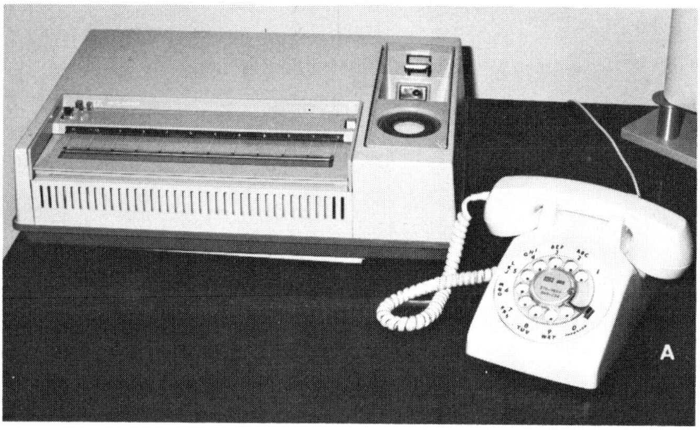

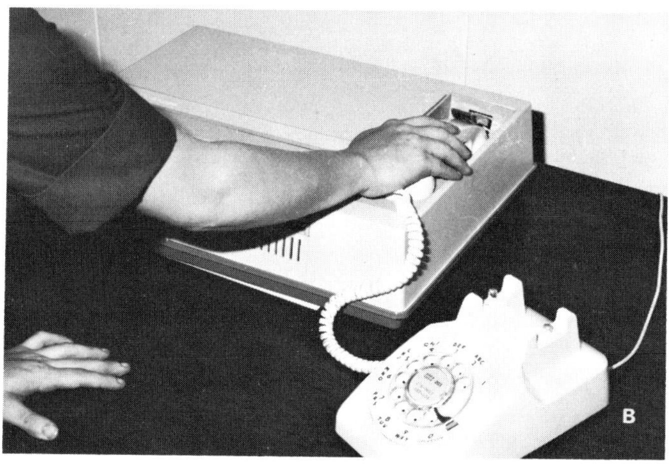

Fig. 8-9. A, The Xerox 400 Telecopier sends and receives a full page of handwritten or printed matter—including dental charts—in a total of six minutes. *B,* Any written or printed matter up to 8 x 10 inches can be transmitted any distance within the country by placing the sheet on a roller inside the machine. The sender notifies the receiver by telephone that he is about to transmit, and they both position the handset on top of their machines. A send button activates document transmission and a receiver button activates copy reception.

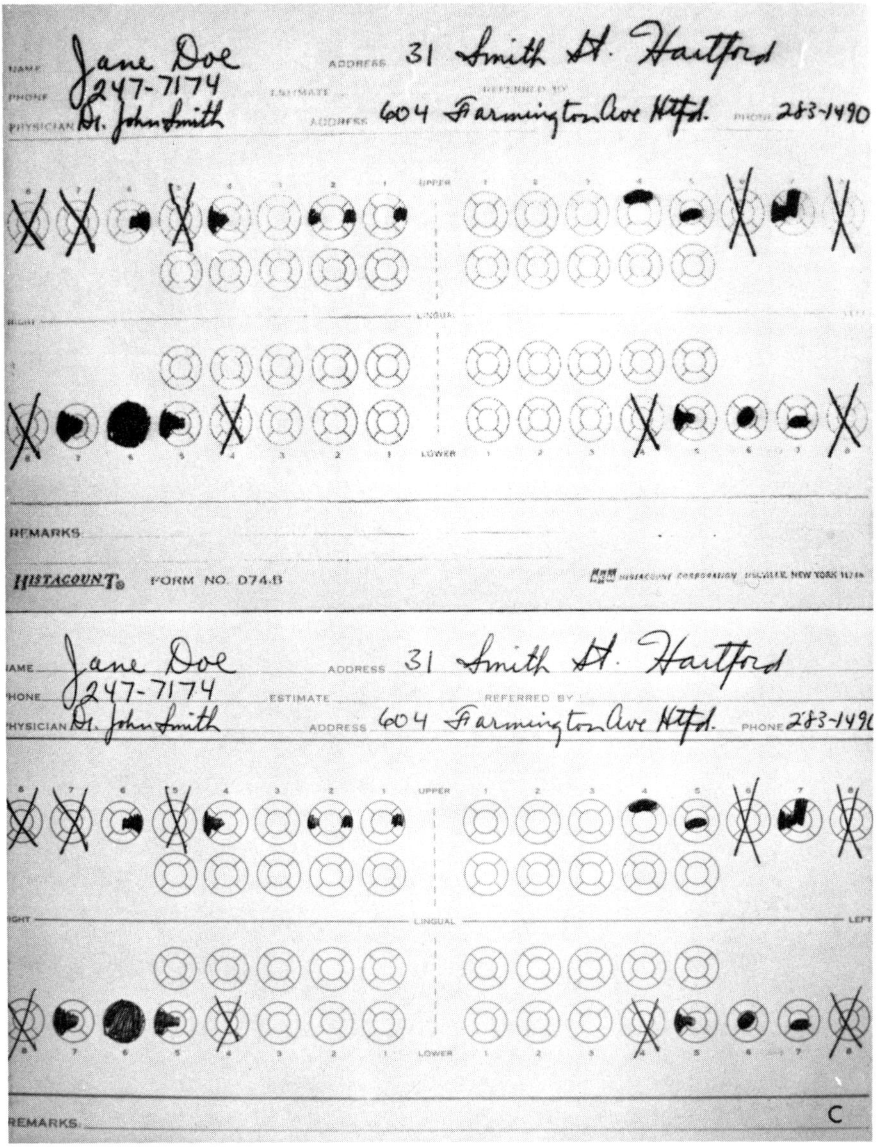

Fig. 8-9. C, Dental chart reproduced by Xerox Telecopier. Bottom chart is the original.

Airline Parcel Service

Some American and foreign airlines offer a service of parcel and document transport on their regularly scheduled planes. The parcel must be delivered to the airport ticket counter, usually by a specified time before departure, and claimed at the airport of destination. Each airline has its own regulations. Among those offering this service are

American Airlines. Priority Parcel Service offered by American Airlines will transport a package only on a direct flight to the point of destination. The package must be at the ticket counter at least one-half hour before flight time. As an example of the rates, the service charge from Hartford, Connecticut, to Los Angeles is $40 prepaid.

Eastern Airlines. Parcel delivery service by Eastern is available only between New York and Washington, D.C., at a cost of $10.

Allegheny Airlines. PDQ (Packages delivered quick) is offered only when the parcel is routed entirely through Allegheny (Fig. 8-10) with no intervening service from other airlines. The minimum charge is $21, including tax, for distances up to 500 miles and $26 for distances beyond that.

British Overseas Airways Corporation. BOAC has a minimum rate of $22 for parcel delivery between New York and London.

Iberia Airlines. The minimum rate charged by Iberia for parcel delivery between New York and Madrid is $24.

SYSTEMS OF DENTAL NOTATION

Over thirty-four different systems of tooth designation are currently in use throughout the world. That the dental profession has not settled upon a single, choice method of recording dental data is relatively inconsequential to the private practitioner accustomed to his own familiar pattern. However, it does pose a problem for the forensic dentist, beset with a multitude of charts and systems of dental notation that he must decipher when studying the antemortem records with which he has been supplied.

Some form of dental notation to designate the teeth and their respective location in the mouth is used in the antemortem diagrammatic dental chart and, usually, in the antemortem written descriptive record. The dentist probably uses the system of notation learned in dental school or, possibly, in the Armed Forces. In the antemortem written descriptive record, which is a verbal description of the treatment rendered the patient, the dentist often makes use of dental abbreviations as well as code symbols for designating the teeth. Occasionally his "personal code" is interspersed in the verbal charting.

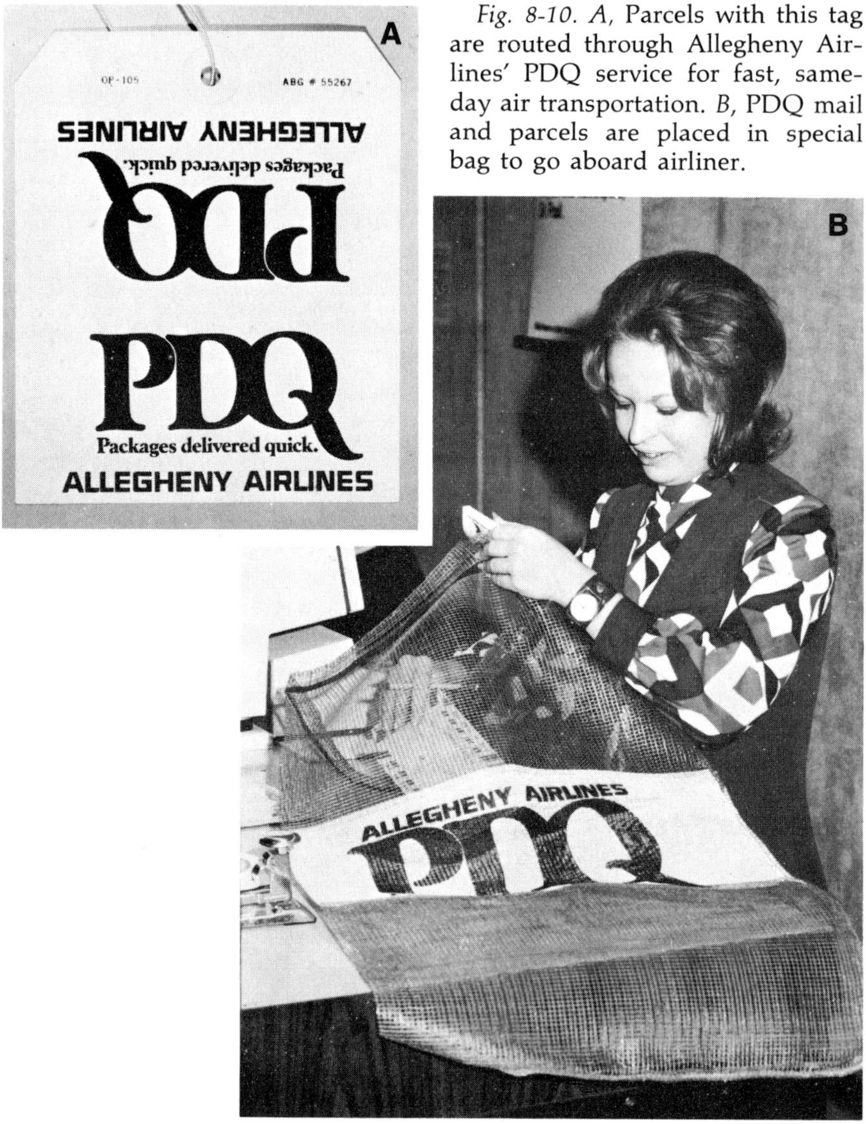

Fig. 8-10. A, Parcels with this tag are routed through Allegheny Airlines' PDQ service for fast, same-day air transportation. *B,* PDQ mail and parcels are placed in special bag to go aboard airliner.

The first step in the perusal of antemortem dental charts is to ascertain the system of dental notation that was used. Since charting is usually done from the viewpoint of the dental examiner as he faces the patient (see Chapter 5), the left side of the dental chart represents the right side of the patient's mouth and vice versa. A few of the better known systems of tooth designation are described below.

Universal System

The Universal System (1-16, 17-32) of tooth designation has been accepted as the standard by the American Dental Association and is now taught in most dental schools in the United States (see pages 88–89).

Palmer's Notation

Up to 1955 the most commonly used method of tooth designation in the United States and parts of Europe was probably Palmer's Notation. Here the mouth is divided into the form of a cross, with the vertical axis representing the midline of the mouth. The teeth are numbered from 8 to 1, starting with the third molar on both sides and continuing toward the midline. Thus, a first incisor is tooth No. 1. The particular quadrant of the mouth in which the tooth is located is represented by a symbol derived from the corresponding quadrant of the cross:

Symbol	*Quadrant of Mouth*		*Symbol*
┘	Upper right	Upper left	└
┐	Lower right	Lower left	┌

The tooth number is placed within the quadrant sign. Thus, 8┘ designates the upper right third molar, and ┌1 the lower left first incisor. In general, the Palmer method of tooth designation is not easily typed or transmitted.

Haderup System

Used extensively in the Scandinavian countries, the Haderup method of tooth designation employs the same numbering system as Palmer's Notation. However, a plus sign (+) is used to designate the upper teeth and a minus sign (−) the lower teeth. The position of the sign, to the right or left of the tooth number, indicates, respectively, the right or left side of the mouth. Thus, −7 refers to the lower left second molar.

F.D.I. Two-digit System

The Federation Dentaire Internationale, an international dental association, advocates a system of tooth designation that employs the same tooth numbers as Palmer's Notation but substitutes for the quadrant sign another number placed before the tooth number:

Quadrant	*Number*
Upper right	1
Upper left	2
Lower left	3
Lower right	4

Accordingly, tooth No. 15 (read one-five) refers to the upper right second bicuspid, and tooth No. 43 (read four-three) to the lower right cuspid. Like the Universal System, it is easily typed and transmitted.

The F.D.I. recently modified its binary numerical code, so that now an odd first number (1,3) refers consistently to the right side of the mouth, while an even first number (2,4) represents the left side of the mouth:

Quadrant	*Number*
Upper right	1
Upper left	2
Lower right	3
Lower left	4

Miscellaneous Systems

The U.S. Armed Forces have adopted the Universal System for dental recording. Previously, the Army used the numbers 8-1, 1-8 to designate teeth in the upper jaw and 16-9, 9-16 for teeth in the lower jaw, with the letter *R* (right) or *L* (left) placed before the number to indicate the side of the mouth. Thus, the lower left third molar is represented by L16. In the system formerly used by the Navy (1-16, 32-17), the upper right third molar is No. 1, the lower left third molar No. 32 and the lower right third molar No. 17.

In still another system of dental notation, a combination of numbers and letters is used to designate the teeth. The numbering system is the same as that in Palmer's Notation. However, letters have been substituted for the quadrant sign:

Quadrant	*Letters*
Upper right	UR
Upper left	UL
Lower right	LR
Lower left	LL

The designation UR6, for example, refers to the upper right first molar.

COMPARING ANTEMORTEM WITH POSTMORTEM RECORDS

After securing the antemortem records, the forensic dentist is ready to continue with the final step that he hopes will culminate in a positive identification of the deceased. Being able to establish a dental identification is contingent upon the availability of usable antemortem records. Without them for comparison, the postmortem information is of limited value.

If there are multiple antemortem records from one or more sources, in order to facilitate comparison with the postmortem record it is recommended that, after ascertaining the system of dental notation used, the forensic dentist, using the Universal System, consolidate all the antemortem information pertaining to a victim onto a Dental Identification Record form (see Fig. 5-5) clearly labeled *Antemortem.* This should probably be considered a requisite procedure in a mass disaster.

In studying the antemortem record, the forensic dentist must be constantly alert to misnomers and discrepancies attributable to tooth migration, uneruption that went unobserved or other oversights. Moreover, it occasionally happens that the wrong tooth is indicated as having been treated or extracted.

Attempting to identify a child by comparing sets of dental charts and x-rays, taken at different times, has inherent problems, for the growth process is constantly changing the oral picture, frequently making it difficult to reconcile the inconsistencies that may appear.

PRELIMINARY STATEMENT OF DENTAL IDENTIFICATION

This certifies that the body of ______________________________
Name of Deceased

was identified by dental means. A complete dental identification report will follow.

____
Dental Examiner

____
Date of Identification

Fig. 8-11. The Preliminary Statement of Dental Identification, issued by the forensic dentist when identity has been established by dental means, expedites the release of the body by the medical examiner.

Furthermore, the similarity in dental charts that can exist from one child to another presents an additional hazard.

Unlike fingerprint identification, dental identification cannot be based on a predetermined number of comparative points, inasmuch as in dental identification certain coincident characteristics are accorded more weight than others. A single antemortem x-ray of a tooth compared with a postmortem x-ray could be the basis for an identification, whereas antemortem and postmortem dental charts showing three or four matching restorations might be regarded as containing insufficient criteria for an identification. If it becomes apparent that there is inadequate evidence upon which to base a dental identification, that information should be made known promptly to the investigating agency.

To resolve the uncertainty of family members and enable the authorities to proceed with appropriate measures, the dentist should endeavor to arrive at a prompt determination of identity or exclusion, in accordance with his professional judgment. Upon making an identification, he should furnish the medical examiner's office with a Preliminary Statement of Dental Identification (Fig. 8-11). The complete dental identification report can follow.

Finally, if summoned to testify in court proceedings, the forensic dentist must be prepared, as a witness expert in his field, to produce, if necessary, demonstrative evidence, such as dental charts, x-rays and photographs, that will (1) verify the findings and substantiate his opinion that the deceased and the missing person are, or are not, one and the same or (2) support his contention that there is insufficient dental evidence on which to base a conclusion.

9 Bite-Marks

Law enforcement agencies use dentistry not only to identify human remains but also to aid in bite-mark investigations. The study of bite-marks is a relatively new aspect of the science of dental identification. Up to now, awareness of the existence of bite-marks has been scant; and their value as dental evidence is still being appraised.

Human bite-marks as incriminatory evidence have been found in foodstuffs, human flesh and other objects. Like fingerprints, the marks made by the human teeth can be a tool for identification. Although historically dental identification predates fingerprinting, the use of bite-mark analysis is just beginning to be recognized, and the procedures are in an incipient stage of development.

Because dentists have limited experience and background knowledge in the evaluation of bite-marks, there is, as yet, no systematic approach to the examination and appraisal of a bite-mark as evidence. Although various procedures have been advocated, each case must be considered on an individual basis, and ultimately, the circumstances peculiar to a case and the facilities available to the forensic dentist will determine the techniques to be employed. Bearing in mind that he may be called upon to substantiate his opinion in legal proceedings, the dentist must proceed cautiously and with the utmost care. In the preparation of court testimony it would probably be prudent for him to consult with knowledgeable colleagues for concurrence relative to his conclusion in a case.

Seen under varying circumstances and resulting from a variety of causes, bite-marks have been found in cases of homicide, robbery, homosexual and heterosexual attack, etc. Although commonly associated with sexual assaults, bite-marks have also been observed in the child abuse syndrome. A bite may be used, moreover, as a defensive weapon (e.g., when the victim bites the assailant). Furthermore, a bite-mark can be unintentionally self-inflicted should an assailant forcefully manipulate the victim's arm against the victim's own teeth. Tooth marks may be left when the teeth come in traumatic contact with another object, as could occur in an automobile accident. Those assorted examples demonstrate the individuality of bite-mark cases and the scrutiny that they demand.

Initial discernment of a bite-mark is no assurance that it will qualify as evidence in a case. Important factors that will determine its validity as evidence are the clarity and quality of the bite-mark—preferably three-dimensional, the presence of distinguishing characteristics apparent upon examination and the results of certain photographic, laboratory and impression techniques. Indistinct tooth marks or other extenuating conditions may preclude its acceptability as a basis for any conclusions.

Case History

A 1½-year-old child, extensively bruised and in a comatose state, was entered into a Bridgeport, Connecticut, hospital by her mother. The child died shortly afterward, with death attributed to internal injuries. The chief medical examiner, reporting evidence that the child had been beaten, summoned the state's forensic dentist to examine what seemed to be human bite-marks that he had observed on different parts of the body during the autopsy.

Although there appeared to be multiple bite-marks, only the mark on the right arm was clear enough to substantiate a finding. From the arch form the dentist concluded that it was a human bite-mark produced by a small mouth. Photographs of the child and of the bite-mark on the right arm were taken by the forensic dentist in black-and-white and color and turned over to the Bridgeport Police.

On questioning the family, the police obtained an admission from a 3-year-old sibling that she had bitten her younger sister during the fatal beating administered by the parents. That concurred with the statement of the dentist that the bite-mark had been produced by a small mouth (Figs. 9-1 and 9-2).

Recognizing a Bite-Mark

Bite-marks frequently go undetected by police officers and, even, pathologists. Generally, the forensic dentist is called into a case when a bite-mark has been noticed by the medical examiner or investigating officer. For bite-marks found in foodstuffs, the suggested procedure is to pour a model in dental stone directly from the impression in the foodstuff, assuming there is a satisfactory reproduction of the facial surfaces of the anterior teeth. Comparing the

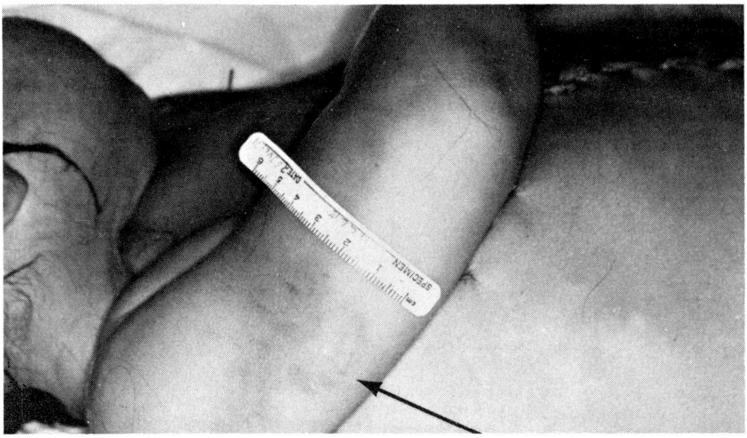

Fig. 9-1. Although commonly considered a sexual manifestation, bite-marks are also encountered in child abuse cases. Bite-mark (*arrow*) on arm of $1\frac{1}{2}$-year-old child was made by 3-year-old sister while parents were beating the victim. Suture marks visible on abdomen are from autopsy procedures.

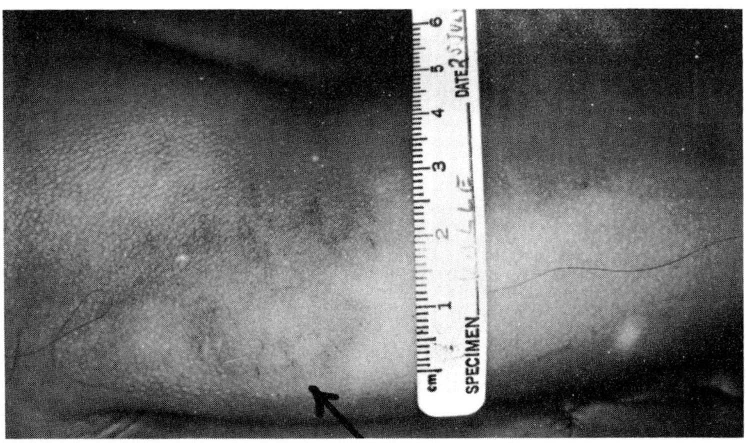

Fig. 9-2. Close-up showing small bite-mark, which appears relatively large on little arm. Arrow points to marks left by lower incisors.

model with the dentition of a suspect might reveal the perpetrator of the bite-mark.

If there is a suspicion that a mark found on a deceased was made by human teeth, the forensic dentist should be summoned promptly and his examination conducted prior to the autopsy: Disturbing the tissues during an autopsy may distort the bite-mark and washing the body may eliminate saliva trace evidence.

Examining the Bite-Mark

As he commences the examination of a mark on a body, the dentist is initially concerned with determining whether it was produced by human teeth. An arch form consistent with that of the human mouth, the teeth of the maxilla distinguishable from those of the mandible and the discernment of characteristic tooth marks would verify the fact that it was a human bite-mark.

The second concern of the dentist is to accurately reproduce the bite-mark for subsequent study away from the body. Accordingly, the mark should be photographed and impressions taken. In addition, an attempt should be made to obtain saliva trace evidence.

Photographing the Bite-Mark. To show size and scale in photographs, a ruler with millimeter scale or a self-adhering millimeter measuring tape should be carefully placed in an unobstructive position near the bite-mark. With quality photographic equipment, black-and-white photographs from different angles should be taken of the bite-mark, the area of the bite-mark and the body in general, including, where possible, anatomical landmarks. At least two close-up shots of the bite-mark should be taken at the proper exposure, and then two additional close-ups—one at one-half stop less and the other at one-half stop more. Using the last two settings compensates for underexposure or overexposure if there was a slight miscalculation initially and, at the same time, affords the chance to pick up other evidence that might not be apparent to the eye. If depressions in the flesh from the teeth can be detected, strong side lighting should be used when the attempt is made to reproduce them photographically.

Color photographs should also be taken to show the hue of the bite-mark, although, because they do not reproduce sharply the details in the lightest areas, they are less effective than black-and-white film for bite-mark study.

Obtaining Saliva Trace Evidence. Since a high percentage of people are secretors, that is, they secrete their blood type factors in other body fluids, such as semen, saliva and perspiration, it may be possible, from saliva found in the bite-mark, to determine the blood group of the perpetrator. Although not sufficient to prove the guilt of a suspect, the evidence may be useful for excluding him.

When an attempt is made to obtain saliva trace evidence, a control should be employed to check the results. A cotton swab dipped into saline solution is used to wash the bite-mark and then sealed in a test tube. A second swab, serving as the control, is dipped into the saline solution and, without coming in contact with the bite-mark, is sealed directly in another test tube. Both tubes are then turned over to a competent forensic laboratory for blood typing.

If no definite results are obtained, it may be due to one of the following: (1) the perpetrator was a nonsecretor, (2) no saliva was left on the bite-mark, (3) saliva trace evidence was removed by prior procedures, (4) a failure in method. Although useful at times, this is not an infallible technique.

Taking Impressions of the Bite-Mark. After saliva trace evidence has been obtained and photographs have been taken, impressions should be made of the bite-mark. At present, silicone is probably the most accurate dental impression material. Manufactured under many different trade names, including Jelcone, Elasticon, Imput, Plastosil, it is available from dental supply companies.

First, free-flowing syringe type silicone should be mixed exactly to the manufacturer's instructions and carefully spread, without voids, over the entire bite-mark area, going beyond the bite-mark itself. When that has set, tray type silicone, which has a thicker consistency, is applied on top and allowed to firm. Finally, to support the silicone and maintain the body contour in the impression material, wet plaster of Paris bandage is added in layers as a backing and allowed to harden before the entire mass is removed from the bite area.

The tissue side of the mass should have reproduced the bite-mark. Since the impression is a negative of the bite-mark, any indentations made in the skin by the incisal edges of the teeth will now be represented by raised areas that can be discerned on the impression under strong side lighting. The raised areas are recognizable apart from artifacts in the impression material.

Examining a Suspect

It is important that a suspect be examined promptly to circumvent the possibility of dental evidence being destroyed through accidental injury or intentional alteration to the dentition. A judicial order authorizing entry into the suspect's mouth should be sought, since the taking of dental impressions of a suspect or the performing of other oral procedures may be considered an infringement of constitutional rights. At the least, written, informed consent of the adult suspect or of the legal guardian of a minor suspect should be obtained before these procedures are commenced.

Taking Photographs of the Suspect. The following close-up and normal views of the suspect should be taken in color and black-and-white:

1. Full face
2. Anterior views of the teeth
3. Incisal edges of the mandibular teeth
4. Incisal edges of the maxillary teeth
5. Front surface mirror views of the incisal edges.

Panatomic-X film for black-and-white pictures and Kodachrome II for color are recommended because they are fine grain films, widely available. Whenever possible, the black-and-white film should be developed before the examination is concluded so that, if it is indicated, additional pictures of the suspect can be taken at that time.

Making Impressions and Models of the Suspect. Impressions of the maxillary and mandibular teeth taken with a fast set alginate impression material will cause minimum discomfort. Before the conclusion of the examination, the impressions should be poured in dental stone and allowed to set. Then, if the models prove to be unsatisfactory, new impressions can be taken at once. In addition, a wax bite should be taken for use in articulating the models.

Studying the Dental Evidence

When the dental evidence is studied, allowance should be made for the fact that a bite-mark is not an exact reproduction of the mouth because of tissue changes coincident with, and subsequent to, the bite. Furthermore, because the entire incisal edge of a tooth may not be situated in the same plane, the complete incisal edge may not always be reproduced. Those portions of the incisal edges of the teeth that extend farther than the others will penetrate more deeply in a bite and produce sharper marks. Teeth situated relatively high in the plane of occlusion might not produce any marks at all. Usually, only the anterior teeth and, possibly, the first bicuspids will produce identifiable imprints in a bite-mark. Following are some techniques that can be employed when the dental evidence is studied.

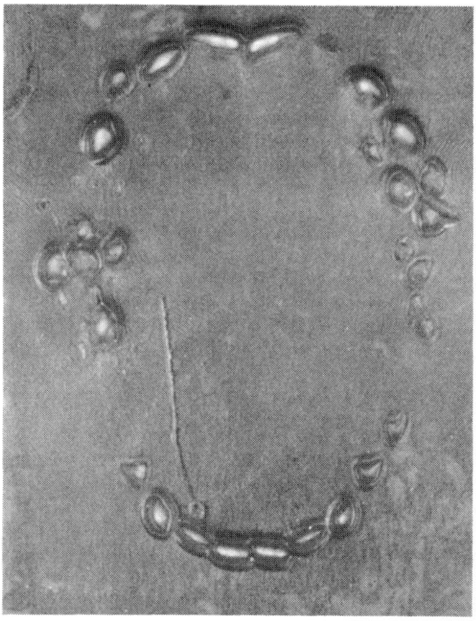

Fig. 9-3. A representation of the tooth alignment in a suspect's mouth can be produced by imprinting the incisal edges of the maxillary and mandibular models into a sheet of pink baseplate wax that has first been placed over white paper. The points of contact will be white where the underlying paper shows through the wax. It may then be possible to align the contact points with the tooth prints in a scale close-up transparency photograph of the bite-mark.

Enlarging Photographs to Scale. Either a millimeter scale ruler or label, like that used in the morgue photographs, should be used as a guide for enlarging 35mm black-and-white photographs of the bite-mark to life-size, yielding a 1:1 relationship, to facilitate comparison with other case materials.

Comparing Models, Photographs and the Impression. Models and photographs of the suspect's teeth are compared to photographs of the bite-mark and to the silicone impression if indentations were present in the bite-mark.

Making Transparencies. The incisal edges of the anterior teeth and the occlusal points of the bicuspids should be outlined on clear acetate that has been placed over the occlusal surfaces of the models. When the transparency is superimposed on a life-size scale photograph of the bite-mark, existing matching points will be evident.

Imprinting Wax. A thin sheet of softened, pink baseplate wax is placed on a sheet of white paper and impressed with the incisal edges of the models, one jaw at a time. The points of contact on the underlying paper will be white where the paper shows through the wax. It is then possible to match the white contact points with the tooth prints seen in a close-up photograph of the bite-mark if points of similarity are present (Fig. 9-3).

Simulating a Bite-Mark on Paper. Onionskin paper and carbon paper,

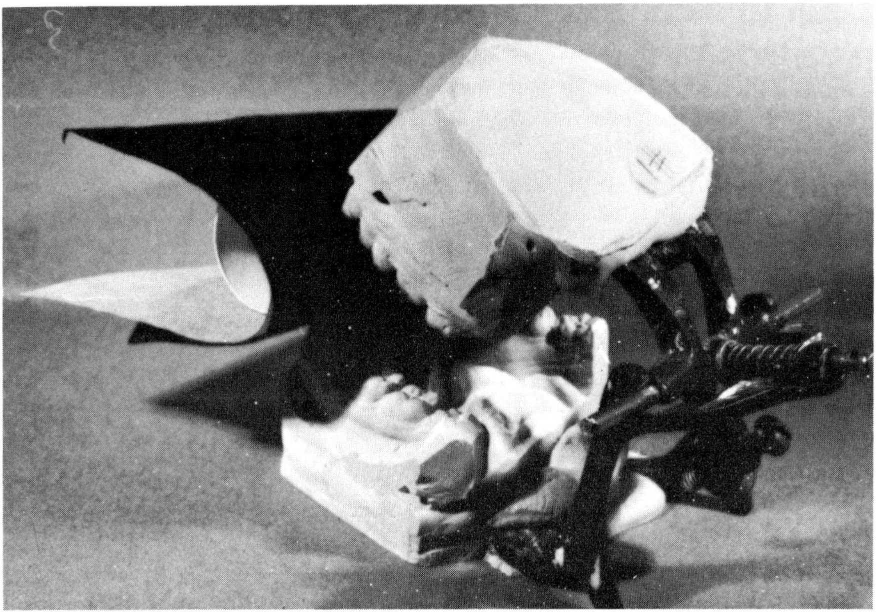

Fig. 9-4. Models of a suspect's teeth are used to produce a bite-mark on paper. Pliable tubing inserted within a folded sheet of both carbon and onionskin papers provides substance for the teeth to clench. Being thin, the onionskin and carbon are readily contoured to the bite.

in that order, are doubled over a short section of wide, pliable tubing without creasing the fold, so that the carbon is on the outside against the onionskin. The articulated models are then closed tightly over the folded, uncreased edge, in the manner of biting (Fig. 9-4). With the models as reference, each black mark produced on the onionskin paper should be assigned a number (Universal System 1-16, 17-32) corresponding to the number of the tooth that made the mark. If the numbered tooth marks match the tooth marks in a scale enlargement of a morgue photograph, the latter, also, can be designated according to the same dental numerical system (see Fig. 9-6). In that way it is possible to identify the individual teeth responsible for the respective marks in the original bite-mark.

Simulating a Bite-Mark on Flesh. A bite produced by the articulated models on the inner part of the forearm of the dentist or a volunteer subject will show the arch formation of the mouth and the tooth alignment of individual teeth. If there is a likeness to the original bite-mark, the reproduced bite can be compared with morgue photographs and might aid in the identification of the individual teeth that had produced the original bite-mark.

The foregoing procedures, which are all within the scope of the practicing dentist, may not be successful in every case. Other procedures that can be used in bite-mark analysis include sophisticated techniques employable by the academician with access to specialized equipment or a forensic laboratory.

Reporting the Conclusion

The forensic dentist, in cooperating with the investigating authorities, should realize the importance of a prompt disclosure of the dental findings. Should he ascertain that the suspect being held could not have been the perpetrator of the bite-mark, it is crucial that the authorities be notified of that fact immediately so that they can reinstitute the search for the culpable party.

If the dental evidence is inadequate to support an opinion (e.g., the bite-mark is indistinct or possesses insufficient distinguishable characteristics), it should be so stated in the report. The techniques used in studying the case should be described and a statement made as to whether the results corroborated or failed to corroborate each other. If the latter, the discrepancies should be noted. In certain instances the forensic dentist may wish to consult with other knowledgeable colleagues.

The dentist presenting actual court testimony but not qualified as an expert witness is restricted to a statement of his observations in the case. The dentist qualified as an expert witness in dental identification may express an opinion based on observations.

THE BITE-MARK KIT

Because a bite-mark kit contains supplies restricted to a specific type of case and is infrequently used, it can be retained separately from the regular dental identification kit. Durable and suitable in size, a 50-caliber Army ammunition case, obtainable at a surplus store, makes a good carrying case for the following items, which are used in bite-mark investigations:

1 container syringe type silicone
1 container tray type silicone
4 rolls plaster of Paris bandage material, (3-inch width)

1 spatula
6 test tubes with stoppers
6 cotton swabs
2 oz. saline solution
2 pairs disposable latex gloves
1 plastic apron
6 self-adhering millimeter scale labels

The manufacturer's instructions must be followed meticulously when the silicone materials are prepared for taking impressions of the bite-mark. Note that silicones have a limited shelf-life. The extra test tubes and swabs allow for multiple bite-marks in a case as well as for accidents in handling.

When impressions are to be taken of a suspect, the dentist can garner from his own office the following supplies:

1 can fast set alginate
1 can dental stone (5 lb.)
1 mixing bowl
1 spatula
1 vibrator
3 upper impression trays (small, medium and large)
3 lower impression trays (small, medium and large)
2 rubber base formers (upper and lower)

Along with either group of items the dentist would also take his photographic equipment and headlight.

Case History

On the night of December 9, 1970, a husky, 17-year-old high school honor student sat at home watching television. The next day four members of his family were dead and he had disappeared.

The discovery of the victims fell to the 44-year-old father returning home that afternoon from work at an industrial plant where he operated the cafeteria. In the living room he found his 14-year-old daughter, nude and strangled, and the nude body of his wife, a registered nurse, who had been stabbed and lay with a hatchet so deeply embedded in her skull that, using both hands, he was unable to dislodge it. Upstairs was his 16-year-old son, who had been hacked to death with the same hatchet, and in her bedroom, his mother-in-law bludgeoned, probably, with the hammer found nearby.

Connecticut's chief medical examiner determined that death had come to three of the victims between four and eight o'clock that morning. The grandmother, still breathing when found was rushed to the hospital, where she died a few hours later without regaining consciousness.

The boy was marked absent from school that day, and a neighbor reported seeing him drive away from the house about 10 A.M. in a tan Chevrolet. Four days later he walked into the Fort Smith, Arkansas police station, the principal suspect in the quadruple homicide. He had traveled there in the tan Chevrolet registered to his now-deceased grandmother. Inside the car were three guns and ammunition that he, upon leaving, had taken from home with the vague idea of living off the land. Denying any recollection of what happened after he last watched television or how he came to Arkansas, he explained that he was prompted to go to a police station because the thought had occurred that his family might be worrying about him.

The murder weapons (hatchet, knife, hammer) were implements belonging to the family and bore no fingerprints. There were no signs of a struggle or of forced entry into the house. The only clue that might connect the suspect to the crime was a distinct, reddish-blue mark on the sister's left breast.

On December 11 the state's forensic dentist was called to the hospital morgue to examine the breast mark. It was a human bite-mark, clear enough for the dentist to distinguish the mandibular and maxillary teeth (Fig. 9-5).

The bite-mark, wider at one end, appeared less oval-shaped than is characteristic of a normal bite. Although there were discolorations indicating where pressure had been applied by the teeth, depressions in the flesh were unable to be detected by the naked eye, probably because of inadequate lighting. Black-and-white and color photographs were taken with close-up and normal 35mm cameras, and an impression was made of the bite-mark.

On December 16, 1970, the state's forensic dentist was requested by the state's attorney, in writing, to take impressions and photographs of the mouth of the suspect, who had just been returned by police escort from Arkansas. Against the advice of the defense lawyer, the suspect, with authorization from his father, voluntarily submitted to having photographs and impressions taken of his mouth, as did the father, who was not a suspect in the case and, later, was excluded positively. The dental procedures, carried out

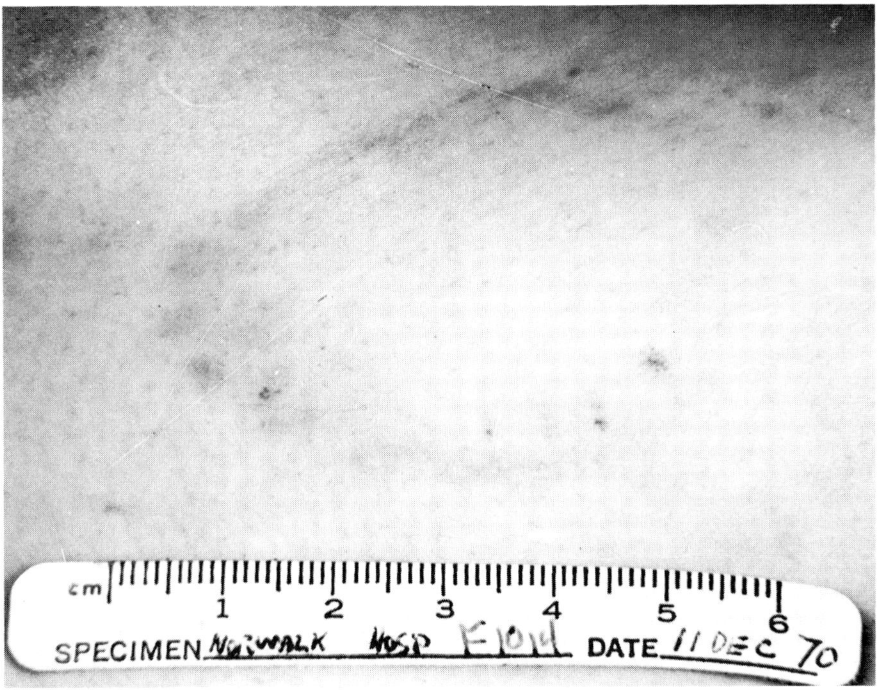

Fig. 9-5. Human bite-mark found on left breast of strangled 14-year-old girl. Although the self-adhering measuring tape is an artifact, it was carefully placed below the bite-mark and does not affect the evidence. Pictures taken initially without a measure demonstrate that the addition of a scale has not effected concealment or in any way altered the evidence. (Figs. 9-5 through 9-7 and 9-9 from Oral Surg., Oral Med., Oral Pathol., *36*:72-78, 1973. Reproduced by permission.)

in the office of the Chief of Police, were made easier by the use of a portable dental headrest, which was attached to a chair.

The photographs of the bite-mark clearly showed (1) the imperfect oval shape of the mark, (2) a differentiation between the upper and lower teeth, (3) a zigzag pattern in the incisal edges of the maxillary teeth, (4) the fairly regular alignment of the lower incisors and (5) the discoloration of the tooth prints on the body.

That the discoloration was slight indicated the bite-mark had been made at, or very close to, the time of death. Had the bite been made a longer time before death, the discoloration would have been greater; had it been made a longer time after death, there would have been less discoloration. Although at the morgue depressions in the bite-mark were not discernible to the naked eye, later, under strong cross-lighting, they were detected as raised areas in the impression.

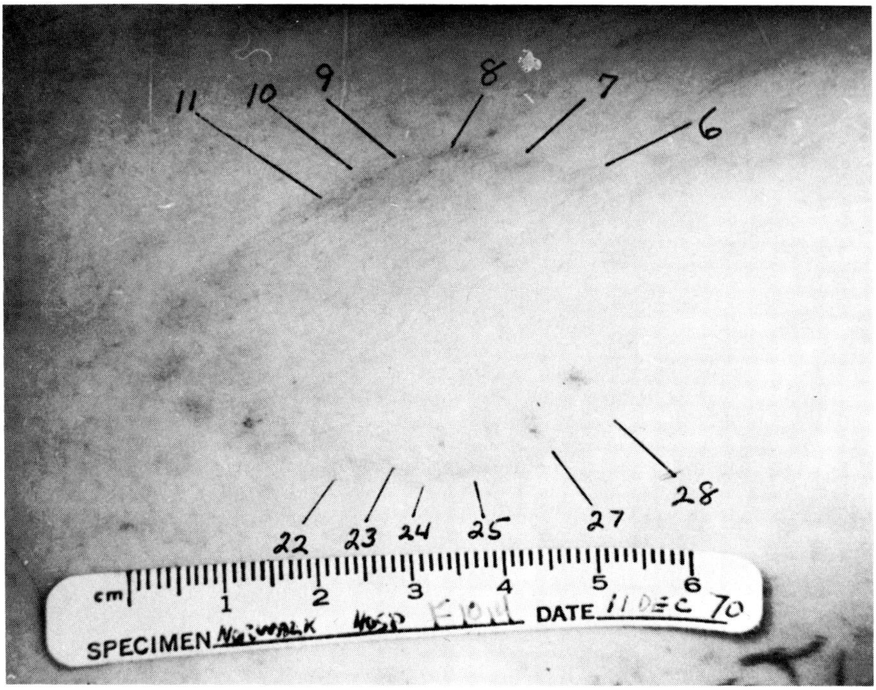

Fig. 9-6. On a photographic enlargement of the bite-mark, the identified tooth marks were designated according to the Universal System (1-16, 17-32). Note zigzag pattern of tooth prints 6, 7, 8, 9 and 10.

In the articulated models of the father, the lower right and upper left second incisors were missing, and the upper first incisors were in alignment. Since the photographs of the bite-mark showed the imprints of all the incisors, with the upper first incisors out of alignment, the bite-mark could not have been made by him.

The techniques described earlier in the chapter were employed in studying and analyzing the dental aspects of the case and served to reinforce each other. All the results were corroborative and there were no inconsistencies.

Critical determinants in the case were the clarity of the bite-mark, the recognizability of twelve tooth prints and their correlation with the respective teeth that had produced the marks (Fig. 9-6), the unusual zigzag pattern of the upper teeth (Fig. 9-7) and the arch formation of the mouth. The bite-mark and the teeth of the suspect yielded well over twenty comparative points. The zigzag pattern of

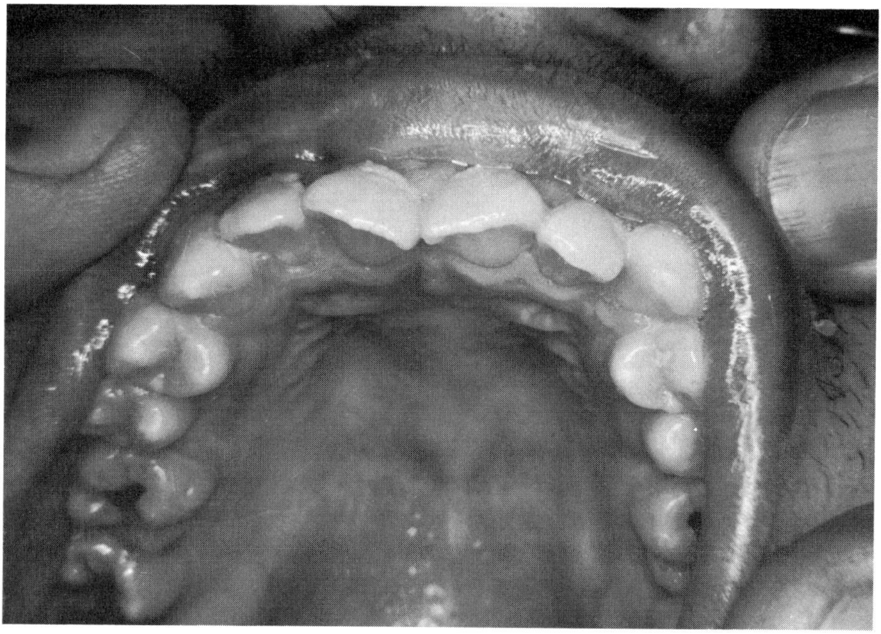

Fig. 9-7. A maxillary incisal view of the suspect's teeth shows the rotation of teeth Nos. 8, 9 and 10 that contributed to the zigzag pattern of the upper anterior teeth, seen, also, in the bite-mark on the victim (See Fig. 9-6).

the maxillary incisal edges and the fairly regular alignment of the lower teeth (Fig. 9-8) were apparent in the photographs and models of the suspect and in photographs of the bite-mark. The imperfect oval shape of the bite-mark was due to the arch formation of the mouth and was duplicated in the bite-marks produced by the suspect's models. Also apparent in the suspect's mouth was a severe Class III malocclusion (protruding lower jaw), a condition that would affect the appearance of a bite-mark produced by such a mouth (Fig. 9-9). From the dental evidence it was determined that the bite-mark had been implanted by the suspect.

At the pretrial hearing, the legality of taking impressions of the mouth of the suspect was upheld, despite the claim of counsel for the defense that dental impressions could be self-incriminating and in violation of constitutional rights. The suspect was tried for first-degree murder in the four slayings on the basis of dental evidence that included photographs, transparencies and articulated models.

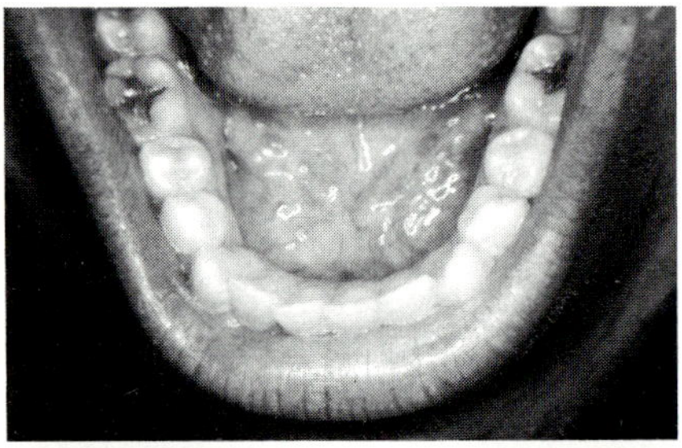

Fig. 9-8. Incisal view of the mandible of suspect shows fairly regular alignment of lower teeth, also seen in bite-mark.

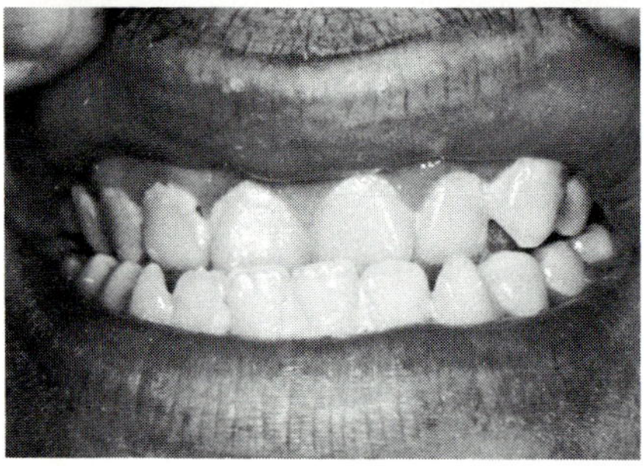

Fig. 9-9. Anterior view of the suspect's teeth in occlusion. The severe Class III malocclusion would have an effect on the appearance of a bite-mark produced by this mouth.

On April 20, 1972, after a $1\frac{1}{2}$-day trial before a three-judge panel, he was found not guilty by reason of insanity and sentenced to a state mental hospital for no more than twenty-five years. During psychiatric examinations he had confessed to the four slayings.

In informal conversation subsequent to the trial, neither the state's attorney nor the counsel for the defense was able to recall any previous American trial in which the prosecution attempted to link a defendant to a murder through tooth marks. Moreover, this is probably the first American court case in which the only incriminating evidence was a bite-mark.

Appendix

SELECTION OF CASES

The procedures used to identify multiple victims by means of the dentition are basically those used to identify a single body. Depending upon the number of victims, however, the services of additional dentists may be needed and supplies in the dental identification kit may have to be increased. Moreover, it is possible that the normal problems of identification may be further complicated by commingled dismemberment or mutilation of the victims.

The Allegheny Airlines disaster of June 7, 1971, exemplifies the techniques employed in handling dental identification in a mass disaster. Although no two disasters are exactly alike, the success of identification is contingent upon (1) skillful recovery of the bodies, (2) careful postmortem dental charting and (3) good antemortem records. The competency in the joint efforts of the investigating officers, forensic dentists and other personnel will influence the accuracy and rapidity with which the individual identifications are accomplished in the aftermath of a mass disaster.

Case History 1

On June 7, 1971, an Allegheny Airlines twin-engine turboprop Convair 580, flying from Groton, Connecticut, enroute to Newport News, Virginia, crashed a mile short of Tweed-New Haven Airport in Connecticut while attempting to make a scheduled 9:52 A.M. landing. Emerging from a low lying fog bank 25 feet above Long Island Sound, the aircraft, carrying 28 passengers and 3 crew members, sheared through high tension wires and three unoccupied beach houses, then exploded and burst into flames. It required the concerted efforts of the fire departments of several towns to extinguish the blaze.

Of the 31 persons aboard, 28 perished in Connecticut's worst commercial airline disaster (Fig. 1). Two passengers and the copilot

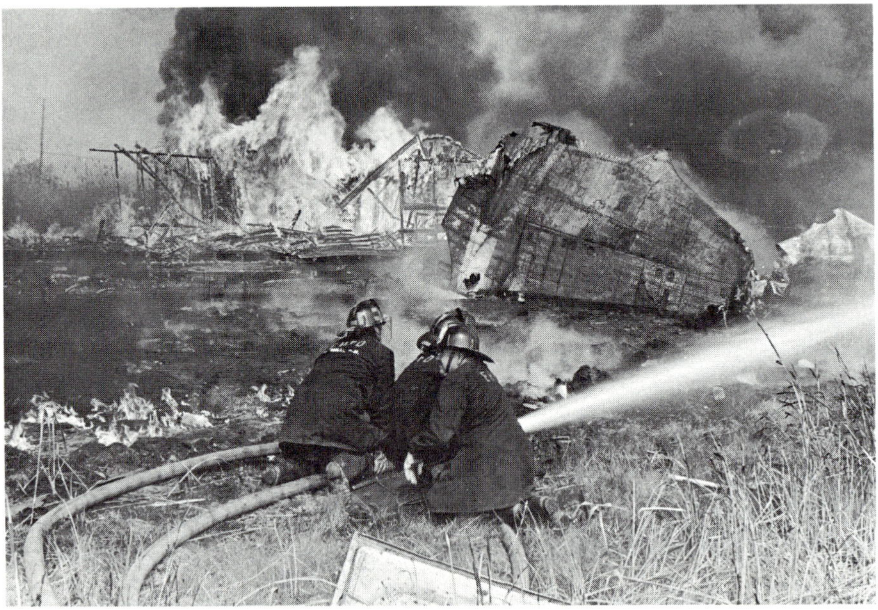

Fig. 1. Burning wreckage of Allegheny propjet that crashed on approach to Tweed-New Haven Airport. To the left can be seen high tension wires and the inflamed beach houses. (*The Hartford Times*)

survived. The copilot was ejected from the plane on impact; a male and a female passenger, suffering burns, managed to escape through an emergency window-exit.

When Connecticut State Police arrived on the scene, only the body of the pilot, in the forefront of the plane and accessible to firemen, had been removed. Later, he was the only victim able to be identified by fingerprints. Before removing the remaining 27 victims, the police photographed and sketched the interior of the aircraft, noting the position of each body and assigning it a number. Each body, along with any personal effects found on it, was then inserted into an individual plastic body recovery bag bearing the same number. Ambulances and hearses transported the victims to Yale-New Haven Hospital. A brief quandary over disposition of the bodies, related to the 90° weather, was resolved by the medical examiner at the scene in favor of Yale-New Haven Hospital, where refrigeration was available. (Where hospital or morgue refrigeration is unavailable, it has been suggested by the FBI that refrigerated trailer trucks be utilized.)

The 27 bodies were burned beyond recognition, and fingerprint identification was impossible. However, the state of Connecticut was in the unique position of having at its disposal a Dental Disaster Squad (DDS), composed of approximately 60 volunteer dentists, organized just two years before by the Connecticut State Dental Association with the cooperation of the Connecticut State Police and prepared to serve in such an emergency. The director of the Dental Disaster Squad was summoned by the State Police Bureau of Identification and asked to assemble the members of the squad for the purpose of identifying the victims by dental means. Permission was granted by the State Chief Medical Examiner and the pathologist of Yale-New Haven Hospital to perform the necessary procedures for dental identification.

Preliminary Examination. Members of the Dental Disaster Squad commenced working about 5:30 P.M. on the day of the accident. They were divided into teams consisting of three dentists each, with an officer from the State Police Bureau of Identification assigned to each team.

The police officers compiled for each victim a file containing the ually from the refrigerator and placed on a table. The dentists were asked to remove jewelry, wallets, fragments of clothing and whatever else they might find on the deceased. These, along with the personal effects recovered at the crash, were recorded by the police officer, in addition to the sex, weight and general size of the body. All personal effects were then retained in a small plastic pouch bearing the same number as the body sack.

The police officers compiled for each victim a file containing the description of the body, the list of personal effects, postmortem dental charts, and, as they were secured, antemortem dental charts and x-rays as well as any other available information. The police worked until midnight, assembling the files and deducing from the data and the passenger manifest possible clues to identity.

Because the bodies had been refrigerated promptly, there was no odor of putrefaction. All had the typical pugilistic pose commonly seen in a burned body (arms drawn up, fists clenched), which is due to the contraction of burned, taut muscles (Fig. 2). The pathologist had determined that all the passengers were alive at impact and death had resulted from the fire. There was no dismemberment or mutilation. Because the tissues of the face and tongue are good insulators, the teeth of the victims appeared to have been protected, except for

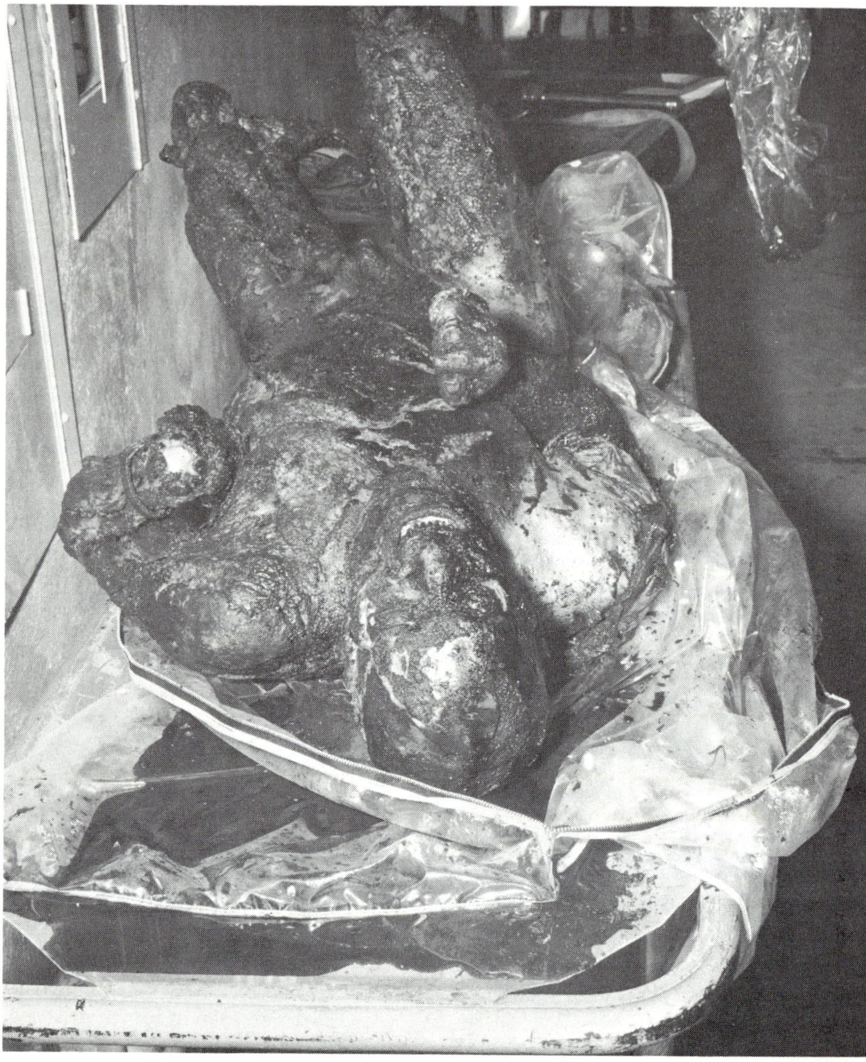

Fig. 2. A burned victim, lying on opened body recovery sack, is seen in characteristic pugilistic pose. Observe watch on left wrist, which may be a clue to identification. (Figs. 2, 3 and 4 courtesy of Journal of Forensic Sciences, *17*:63, 1972)

the facial surface of the anterior teeth. On observation, the lips of the victims had the aspect of being slightly parted.

Dental Procedures. Because the burned facial muscles severely restricted the opening of the oral cavity, unremedied by incisions in the facial tissue, it was deemed necessary to resect the mandible to gain access to the mouth. With a No. 20 blade scalpel, an inverted *V* incision was made on each side of the mouth. When the tissue flap was pulled back, the bone of the mandible became clearly visible. A Stryker autopsy saw was then used to cut through the left and right sides of the mandible beyond the most posterior teeth. Cutting into the lingual mandibular border with a scalpel and freeing all muscle attachments enabled the mandible to be easily lowered, permitting an unobstructed view of both the maxillary and mandibular dentition.

Each team of three dentists was instructed to record on the postmortem dental chart for each victim teeth that were missing, caries, restorations and their material, bridgework and other prosthetic appliances and any unusual conditions related to tooth shape, alignment, arch formation, etc. The Universal System (1–16, 17–32) of tooth designation was used on a diagrammatic chart. As the first dentist to examine the mouth called out his observations, they were recorded on the chart by another member of the dental team (Fig. 3). A third dentist then made his examination. Finally, as the recording dentist read aloud the charting, the three reexamined the mouth, resolving any discrepancies that might have occurred. The fact that the postmortem charts, when compared with antemortem x-rays and records, appeared to be error free was attributed to the triple-check system and the scrupulous attention exerted.

By 11 P.M., 25 bodies had been examined. The 25 postmortem dental charts were taken across the street to the library of Yale-New Haven Hospital, where Xerox copies were made. Later, Xerox copies were made of the antemortem charts, and the antemortem x-rays were reproduced on photographic film (Fig. 4) so that the original antemortem charts and x-rays could be turned over to the U.S. Federal Bureau of Investigation in accordance with their request.

The passenger manifest listed two young children in the same family whose recognizable body size was acceptable for identification. The body of one, a 6-month-old baby, was recovered in proximity to its mother, and the body of the other, a 2-year-old, was found near the body of the father.

The next evening two of the dentists who had participated in the examinations the preceding day, accompanied by two additional volunteers from the Dental Disaster Squad (a total of 18 Connecticut dentists took part in the investigation) returned to Yale-New Haven

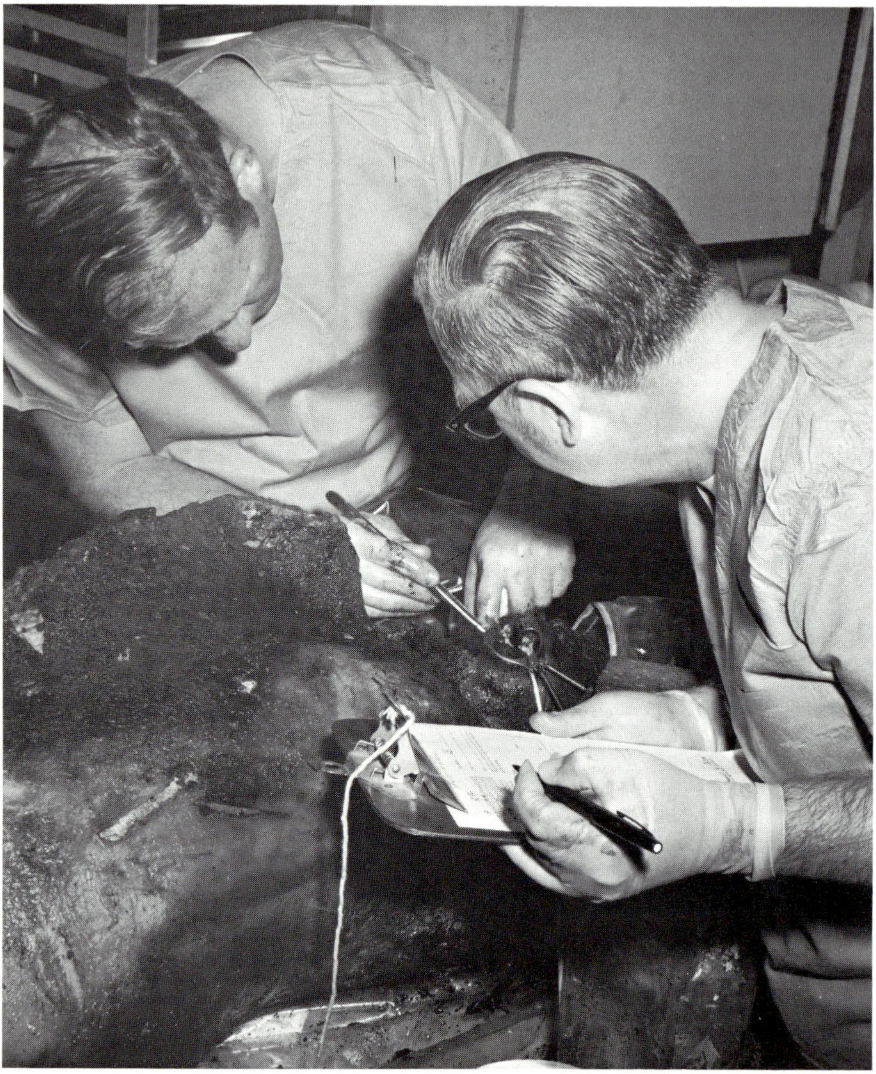

Fig. 3. Members of a dental team examining and charting the dentition of a victim. State Police officers recorded personal effects and other nondental information.

Hospital for the purpose of comparing antemortem and postmortem records. By 11 P.M. that night, based on the records that had been obtained, 21 of the 25 bodies had been identified. Records on the remaining victims continued to arrive. By the following evening all 28 bodies had been identified.

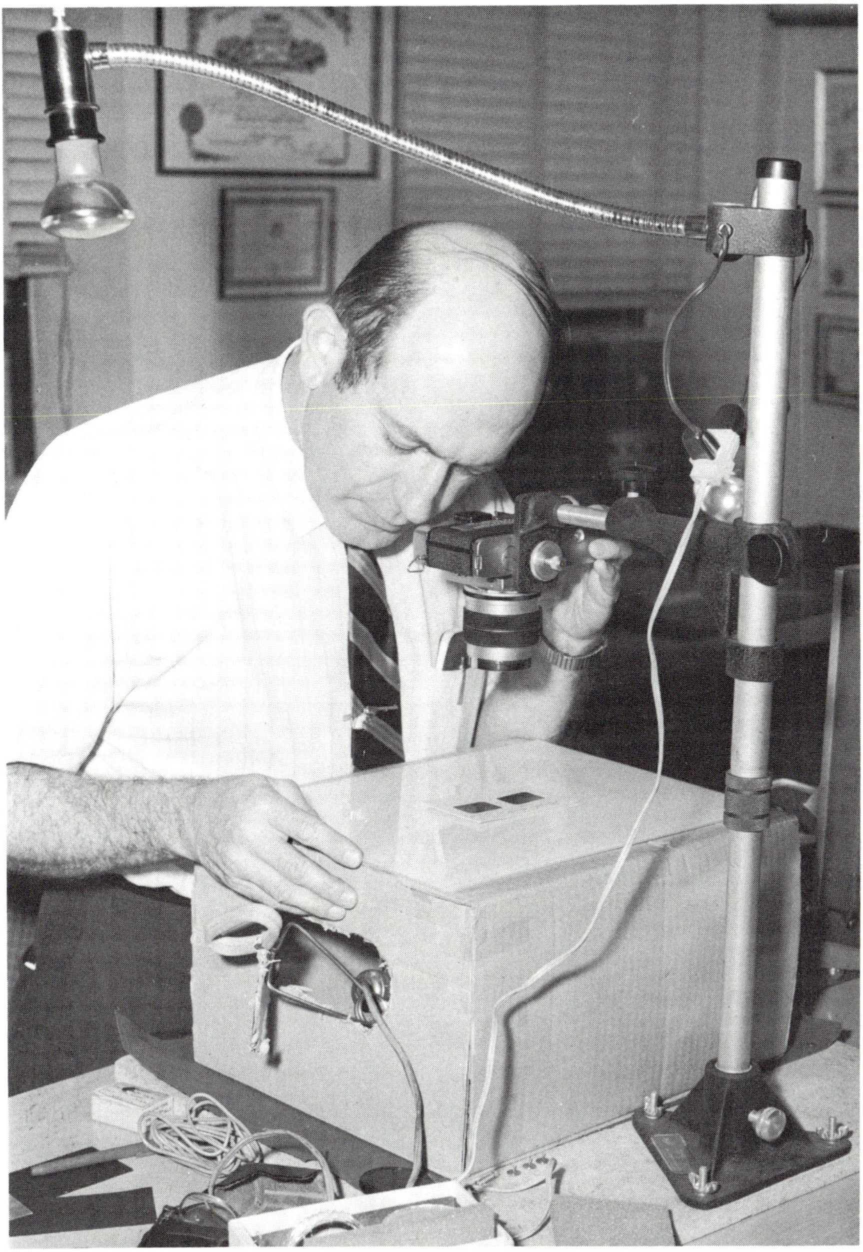

Fig. 4. With the use of an extension tube placed between the lens and body of a 35mm Topcon camera, antemortem x-rays are photographed on black-and-white film, from which multiple prints can easily be made. Lighting source is a photoflood bulb enclosed in a cardboard box and covered with opal glass.

Antemortem Records. Antemortem records were procured by the police, FBI, airline officials and members of the Dental Disaster Squad. They consisted of diagrammatic charts, written charts, detailed verbal descriptions and periapical, bite-wing and panoramic x-rays. (It was the opinion of the examiners that bite-wing and panoramic film were more easily read, for comparison purposes, than periapical x-rays.) In a few cases it was necessary for dentists of the squad to obtain a detailed oral description of the antemortem chart and x-rays over the telephone from the victim's dentist. That was considered the least satisfactory, but nevertheless an acceptable, method of establishing identity. The charts and x-rays, arriving subsequently by mail, substantiated the identification.

The dental records of the stewardess, who was single, were difficult to locate. Allegheny Airlines, like the other major air carriers, does not maintain dental records (charts or x-rays) of its flight personnel. (The practice of retaining dental information on people in hazardous occupations is referred to as "precautionary registration.") After numerous long distance telephone calls, the dental records were finally traced to a Pennsylvania dentist, who promptly transmitted over the telephone a complete charting of the mouth, including a detailed description of a microbond fixed bridge that was an important factor in her dental identification.

Four sets of Navy antemortem dental charts, all different, were supplied for one of the victims, the discrepancies being due to the incorrect designation of teeth that had migrated into spaces left from extractions. This case demonstrates the hazard of having to depend on dental charts, without antemortem radiographs, for identification. Fortunately, the Navy also furnished x-rays, and identification was predicated on the antemortem x-rays.

A soldier with perfect teeth, no caries or restorations, was congenitally lacking the upper second incisors. The distraught father was reluctant to accept the fact that the body was that of his son. However, an Army panoramic x-ray clearly revealed the unusual dental condition, so that the identification was indisputable.

The family of another victim requested, for religious reasons, that the body be identified immediately and released for burial. To comply, the FBI had the antemortem dental records transmitted that same day from Washington, D.C., by Xerox Telecopier. Although that was the first body to be identified by the Connecticut Dental Disaster Squad, it was not released until all the victims had been

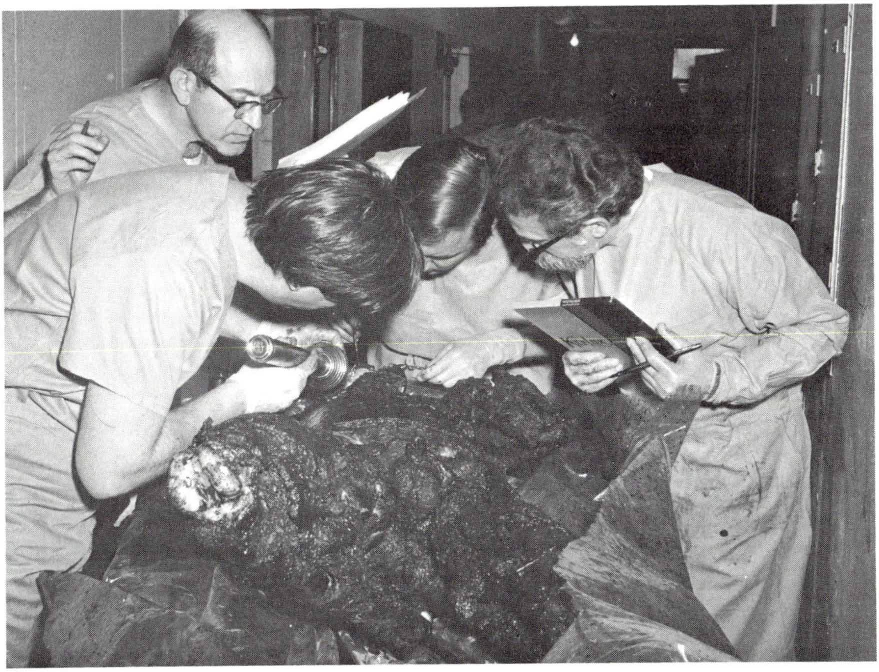

Fig. 5. Dental examination being conducted by team of three Squad members in narrow, poorly lit corridor of basement undergoing remodeling at Yale-New Haven Hospital. Insufficient lighting from bare bulbs strung overhead on temporary, exposed wiring was supplemented by 5-cell flashlight loaned by State Trooper. Scrub suits and rubber gloves were supplied by hospital. Squad Director is collecting completed postmortem charts from dental team. (Connecticut State Police)

identified. (To minimize errors in identification following a mass disaster, no body should be released until the identification procedures for all the victims have been completed.)

Problems and Solutions. As the basement of Yale-New Haven Hospital was in the midst of being rebuilt, physical working conditions for the dentists were poor. Most of the dental examinations were conducted in the restricted space of the corridor, outside the morgue (where the autopsies were being performed), under temporary lighting strung overhead on exposed wiring. The State Police troopers loaned the dentists their 5-cell flashlights to help compensate for the inadequate lighting (Fig. 5).

At that time, the Connecticut Dental Disaster Squad did not have headlights or a Stryker autopsy saw in the dental identification kit. The autopsy saw, a necessity in a mass disaster, was made available by the hospital. A 150-foot heavy-duty extension cord with multiple outlets would have been useful as an electric source for additional illumination and for photographic equipment. Also demonstrated was the desirability of a telephone committee to notify those dentists whose services were needed, thus allowing the Squad director to depart without delay for the scene of the accident, and for some type of badge or identity card for the Squad dentists, who at first experienced difficulty gaining admittance to the hospital.

This initial effort of the Connecticut Dental Disaster Squad probably marks the first time that an organized group of volunteer dentists, prepared to assist in the event of a mass disaster, was summoned into service by law enforcement officials. The unqualified success of the endeavor encourages the formation of similar forensic dental groups throughout the United States and other parts of the world.

* * * * *

In cases of suicide, as in other questions of identity, dental identification is resorted to only when other methods of identification cannot be used. If the victim selected a solitary place for his ultimate act, the body, when finally discovered, may be extensively decomposed, depending upon climatic factors such as temperature, wind, humidity, etc. Because the suicide victim frequently has a history of mental illness, a mental or general hospital may be a source for antemortem dental records.

Case History 2

A hiker came upon the remains of a human being hanging from a tree (Fig. 6) in the woods near Barkhamstead, Connecticut. The police were notified, and on authorization from the medical examiner, the victim, apparently a suicide, was cut down and removed to a mortuary.

The partially decomposed body had mummified, attributable to climatic conditions and the absence of flies (Figs. 7 and 8). Papers found in the victim's clothing contained the name of a missing man who, it developed, had a long history of mental illness. Identification was based on the comparison of postmortem dental records with antemortem dental records supplied by the State Mental Hospital.

* * * * *

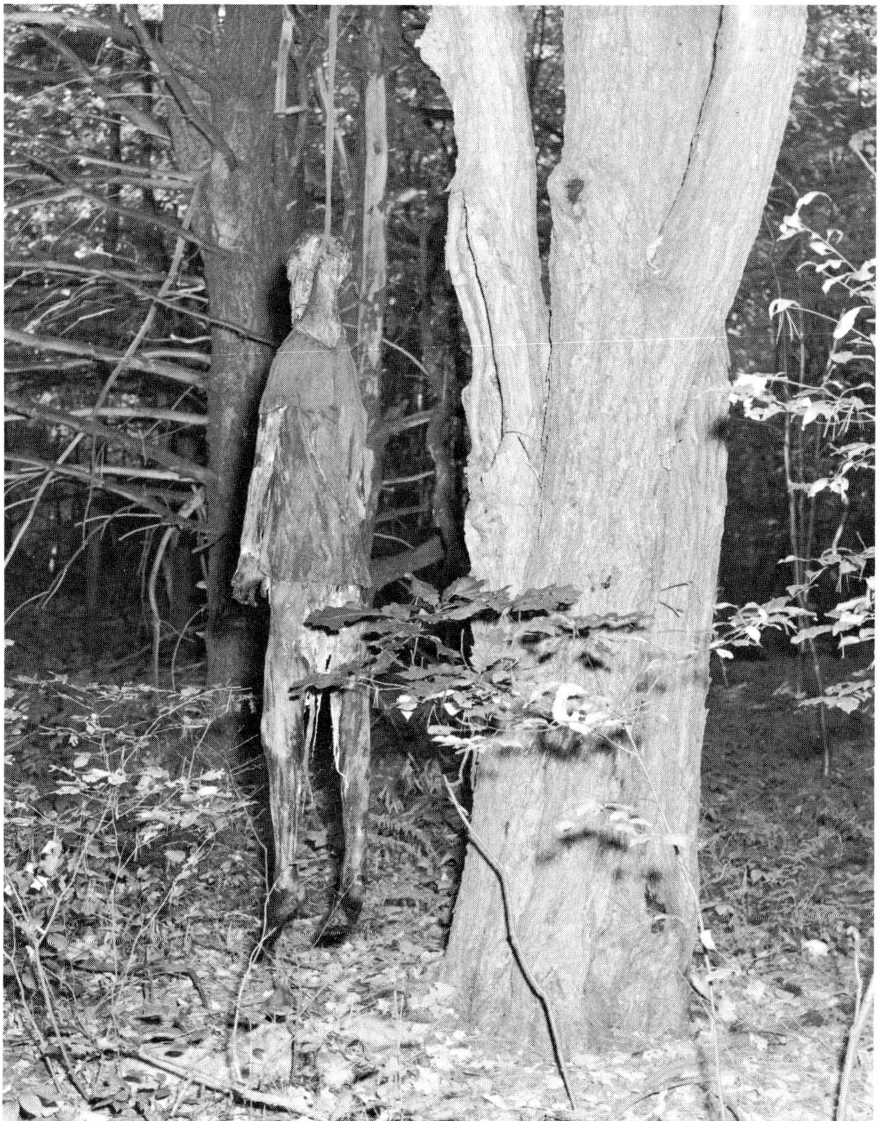

Fig. 6. Suicide victim found hanging from tree. Neck was stretched by the rope. (Connecticut State Police)

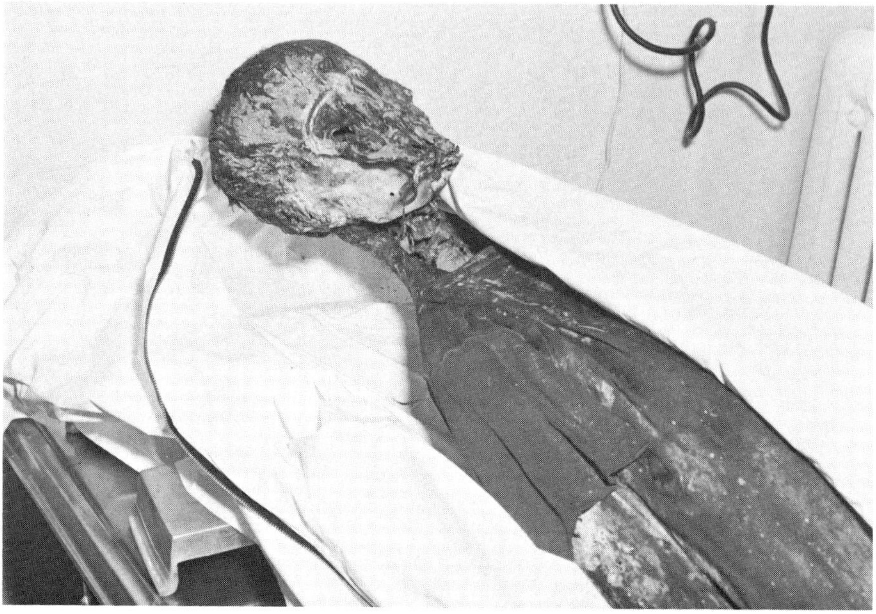

Fig. 7. Climatic conditions had caused the body to mummify. (Connecticut State Police)

Attempts by persons to fraudulently claim an unidentified body are not uncommon. Pending estate settlement or resolvement of legal obstacles to remarriage, they will sometimes fraudently claim an unidentified body as a way out of their personal predicament. Others may have in mind the express purpose of viewing a dead body (necrophilia) or the hope of obtaining the insurance payment.

Police departments have ways of uncovering such subterfuge. One device employed is to ask, for example, "Did your uncle have a long scar across his neck and the lower part of his face?" When the purported relative responds affirmatively to the leading question, he is then informed that this could not be the missing relation.

It is assumed, however, that in the following case the claimants acted without ulterior motives.

Case History 3

After extinguishing a fire in a vacant three-story building slated for demolition, the firemen discovered, propped up against the wall in the corner of a room, the charred remains of an alcoholic vagrant, who had probably caused the fire by careless smoking. There were

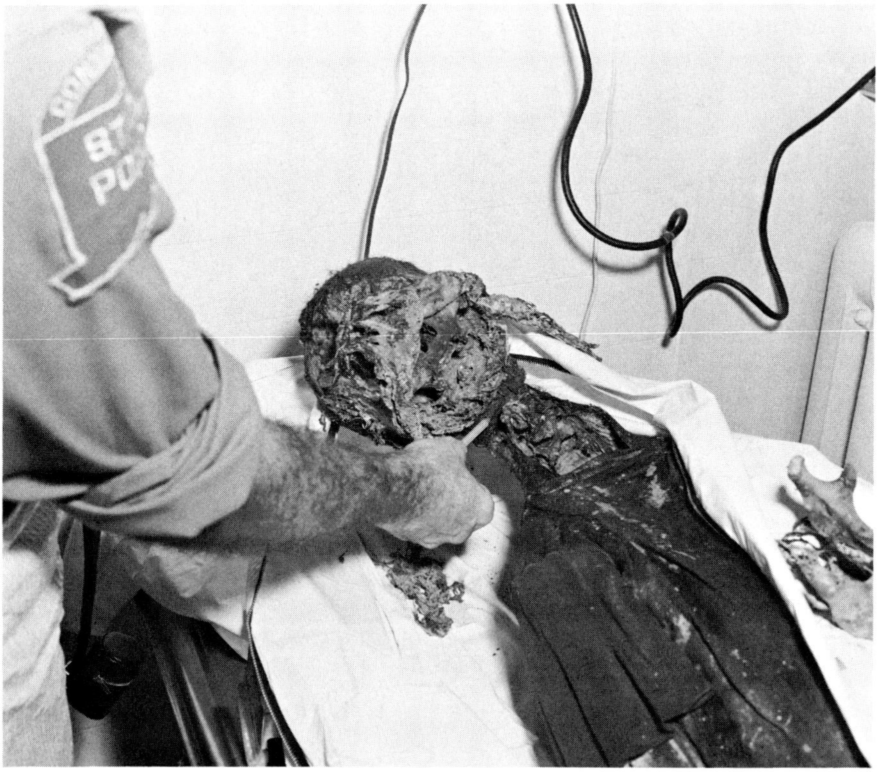

Fig. 8. Leathery skin was easily cut away with scissors and scalpel, freeing mandible for examination. Detached mandible is on table to right of body. Pencil points to rope still tied around victim's neck. (Connecticut State Police)

no specific clues to identity on or near the body. However, it was noticed that the victim had a glass eye (Fig. 9). The body was taken to a mortuary, and the forensic dentist was summoned.

Two families, having read the newspaper story, came to claim the victim. One family reported a missing uncle with a left glass eye. However, the body had a right glass eye.

The other family, whose missing relative had a right glass eye, believed he had never been to a dentist. The chief of detectives supplied the forensic dentist with the information that the missing man had lost an eye in a logging accident in Tuskegee, Alabama, and had been fitted with an artificial eye in the Veterans Administration Hospital in Montgomery.

Aware that patients in a Veterans Hospital frequently go through

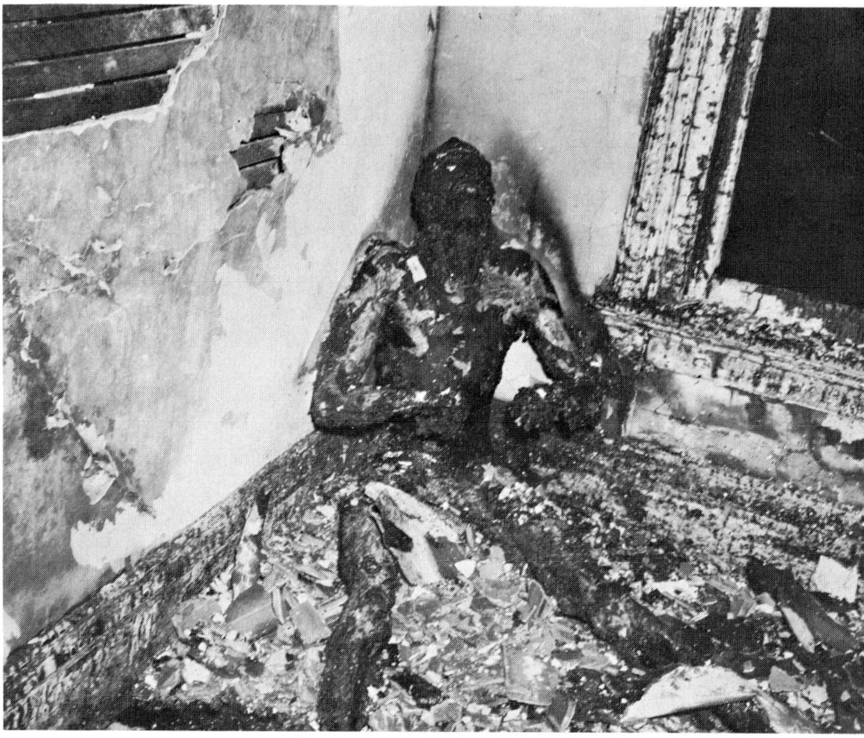

Fig. 9. Vagrant burned in fire has arms in the typical pugilistic pose often seen in a burned body. Artificial right eye is visible in photograph. (Hartford Police Department)

the dental clinic, the forensic dentist telephoned the Alabama V.A. Hospital to inquire about dental records, which were located in the man's file. The V.A. dentist reported that antemortem records showed no caries or restorations, but the lower second and third molars were missing.

Resection of the mandible was necessary to examine and chart the mouth. Identification was based on the matching antemortem and postmortem dental charts and the coincidental right glass eye of the victim and the missing person.

* * * * *

Bullets and, especially, shot-gun pellets can splinter or fragmentize the jaws and dentition. Where such is the case, it may be necessary to search the recovery site for pieces of jaw and teeth that were not retrieved with the body. Furthermore, as demonstrated below, the

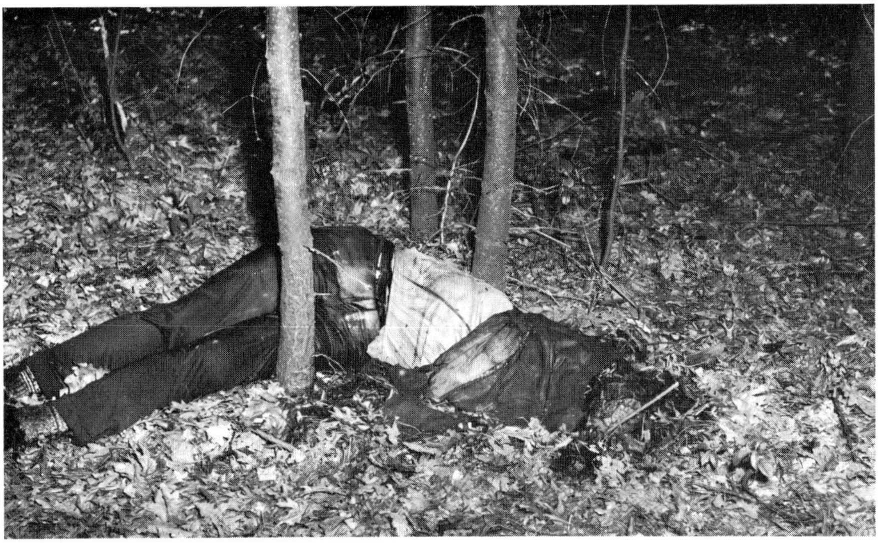

Fig. 10. Body found in woods by police after anonymous telephone call. (Connecticut State Police)

extent of decomposition in a body is not always a reliable indicator of the time of death, since extreme heat and humidity and the presence of maggots can accelerate the deterioration process.

Case History 4

An anonymous telephone call directed the State Police to an extensively decomposed body that had been dumped in a wooded area in Somers, Connecticut (Fig. 10). Judging from the amount of decomposition that had taken place, the pathologist examining the body in the hospital morgue estimated death had occurred at least eight weeks before (Fig. 11).

The victim had been shot through the head four times with a 45-caliber pistol. One of the bullets, having entered the right side of the mandible and crossed upward at a 45° angle, had removed a large portion of the left side of the maxilla. In the victim's pants pocket was found an expired driver's license bearing the name of an ex-convict released from State Prison only thirteen days before, which did not correspond with the time of death set by the pathologist.

The forensic dentist requested the prison dental records. Although the upper left anterior and posterior teeth were not present in the

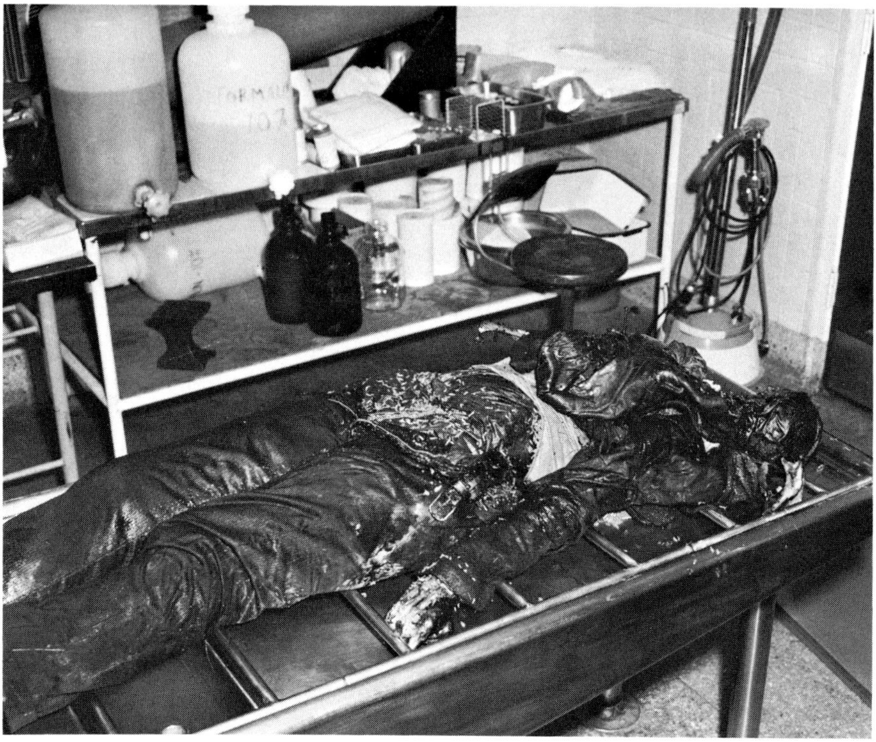

Fig. 11. Extensively decomposed body in morgue. Small, whitish objects in lower abdominal region are maggots (fly larvae), often found in decaying matter during warm weather. (Connecticut State Police)

skull, the remaining teeth, compared with the antemortem dental record, constituted sufficient evidence on which to base a positive identification of the ex-convict. In addition, from the dental records the dentist inferred that nine teeth had been torn from the skull by the force of the bullets. Searching the recovery area the next morning for dental remains, the State Policemen located the nine teeth and the missing jaw fragment.

The extreme heat and humidity of that particular time period and the activity of rodents and maggots probably accounted for the body's advanced state of decomposition.

* * * * *

Even though an edentulous victim wearing plastic dentures has been severely burned, the dentures are likely to be recovered, for the facial tissues are excellent insulators. Likewise, because the newer styrene material is less easily fragmented, it is possible for recently

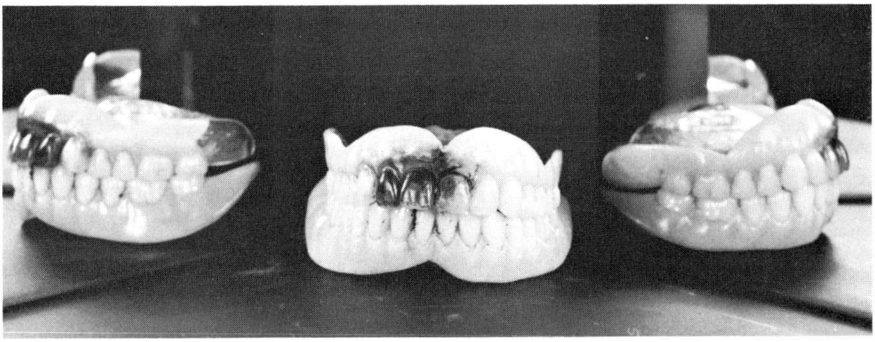

Fig. 12. Full upper and lower acrylic dentures removed from mouth of victim burned beyond recognition. Observe minimal burn damage to dentures, which were the basis for the identification. Three-sided photographic view was produced with two stainless steel mirrors positioned at 45° angles to the camera.

constructed styrene dentures to be recovered even where mutilation of the victim has occurred. Oftentimes much information helpful in identification can be gleaned from, particularly, the anterior denture teeth of the maxilla, since they are manufactured in a greater variety of shapes and sizes than the other denture teeth.

Case History 5

A small, imported, French car with a rear engine had stopped for a signal light on the Berlin Turnpike in Berlin, Connecticut. Approaching from behind, the driver of a trailer truck failed to observe the stoplight and crashed into the car. It immediately burst into flames, entrapping the three occupants.

Berlin firemen, after extinguishing the flames, removed two bodies from the front seat and one from the back. The police ascertained the owner of the car from the license plates and, also, that its occupants at the time were the owner, his wife and a female friend of the family.

Because the bodies were burned beyond recognition, the forensic dentist was summoned to make the identifications. According to the antemortem dental records, the friend wore full upper and lower dentures. The body recovered next to the man, who had been driving the car, was not that of his wife but of the friend, whose dentures had suffered minimal damage despite the extensive destruction to the body (Fig. 12). The dentures matched the descriptive facts contained in the antemortem dental record: Dentsply porcelain teeth,

20° posteriors, clear palate in the upper denture, two repairs in the lower denture. Thus the dentures constituted an acceptable basis for identification of the edentulous victim.

Satisfactory antemortem dental evidence for the two other victims, who had natural teeth, was difficult to obtain, inasmuch as the husband, an x-ray engineer, had not permitted x-rays to be taken of himself or his wife for the last ten years. Consequently, the records of the local dentist failed to include sufficient data to make an identification. Finally, the victims' former dentist, who had retired to Florida eleven years before, was located. Fortunately, he had retained most of his dental records intact and was able to supply the forensic dentist with x-rays, enabling him to make a positive identification of the burned couple.

* * * * *

Jewelry, wearing apparel and other personal effects found on a deceased, although not the basis for an identification, may act as clues to identity. Wariness is called for, however, since personal effects as clues can also be unreliable and misleading, as demonstrated in the following case.

Case History 6

Witnesses reported seeing a new 1967 automobile speeding by with sparks shooting from the rear. Despite the fact that the brake lights were on, indicating the driver was attempting to stop, the speed seemed to be quickening, and there were reports of a woman's screams issuing from the car. The car sped off a ramp leading from the incompleted expressway, smashed into an intersection wall and burst into flames (Fig. 13).

The firemen were unable to free the driver until fifteen minutes later (Fig. 14), when the body was removed to the morgue at Hartford Hospital. Through the license plates and car registration, the victim was tentatively identified as a bank director and the wife of a prominent local attorney. However, the initials engraved on the rings removed from her fingers did not coincide with the initials of the presumed victim.

The state's forensic dentist was summoned when visual identification was not possible. The face had not been totally burned and resecting the jaws was not indicated. Cuts at the commisures of the mouth provided sufficient access for examining and charting, and identification was made by comparing antemortem and postmortem dental records. It was learned that the victim had been wearing family

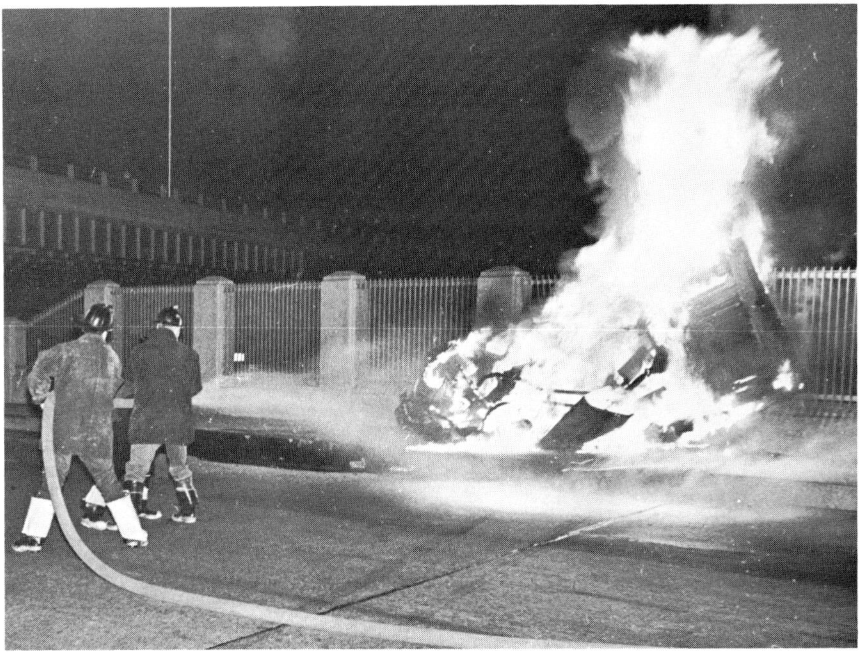

Fig. 13. Firemen fighting twenty-foot flames of burning car. Victim was trapped inside. (*The Hartford Times*)

jewelry, which fact accounted for the discrepancy in the initials. Subsequently, an extensive investigation was conducted to determine whether the accident had been caused by a malfunctioning in the automobile.

* * * * *

Another aspect of forensic dentistry, dental fraud, unexpectedly came to light in what, supposedly, was an uncomplicated dental identification of an apparent murder victim.

Case History 7

An anonymous telephone call led the police to a headless skeleton (Fig. 15) lying under a pile of rocks off the Merritt Parkway, near Stamford, Connecticut. It was the same area where a Negro prostitute had been reported missing and, several months before that, two other Negro prostitutes, friends of the missing woman, had been found strangled by their bras. Both had been identified visually at the time of recovery of the bodies. The three women came from the same city and had mutual friends.

The skeleton was intact except for the skull, which was recovered

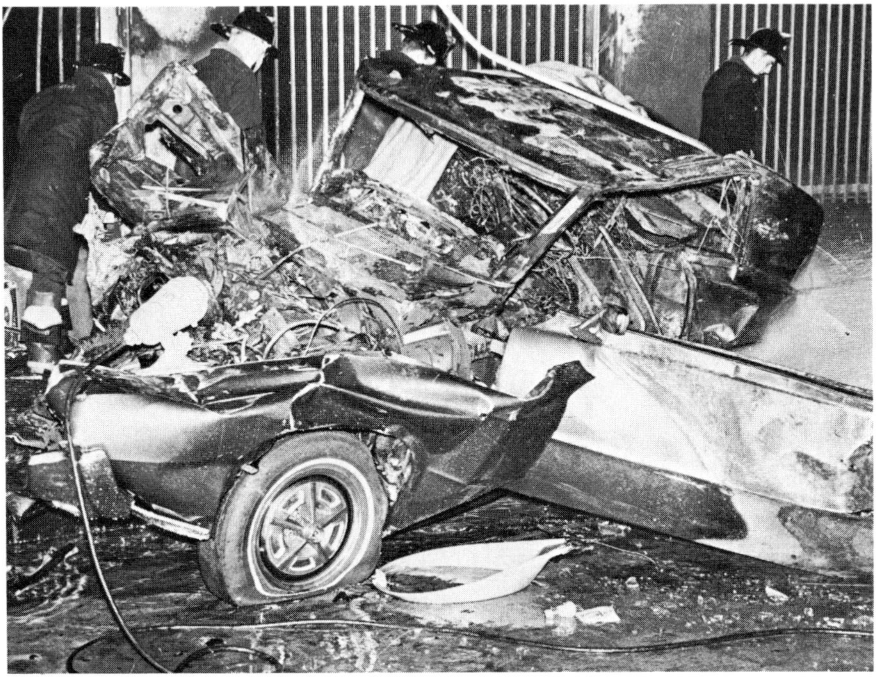

Fig. 14. Victim removed from demolished car was burned beyond recognition, necessitating identification by dental means. (*The Hartford Times*)

a few days later. It had been crushed postmortem and the pieces scattered. The police theorized that the skeleton was that of the missing black woman.

The victim's dentist, whose name was supplied by the family, had no x-rays and surrendered his dental records with obvious reluctance. When the pieces of skull were assembled and the mouth was charted, it was discovered that certain fillings recorded on the antemortem chart were not present postmortem. The discrepancies precluded a positive identification.

The missing woman had been a welfare recipient, and from a check of state welfare records, it appeared that the dentist had received payment for work not evidenced in the skull. Welfare files disclosed the name of another dentist who had treated her, unknown to the family. His x-rays, corresponding with the postmortem dental examination, enabled an identification to be made (Fig. 16). One could infer that the first dentist had billed the state for dental services he had not performed—an apparent case of dental fraud.

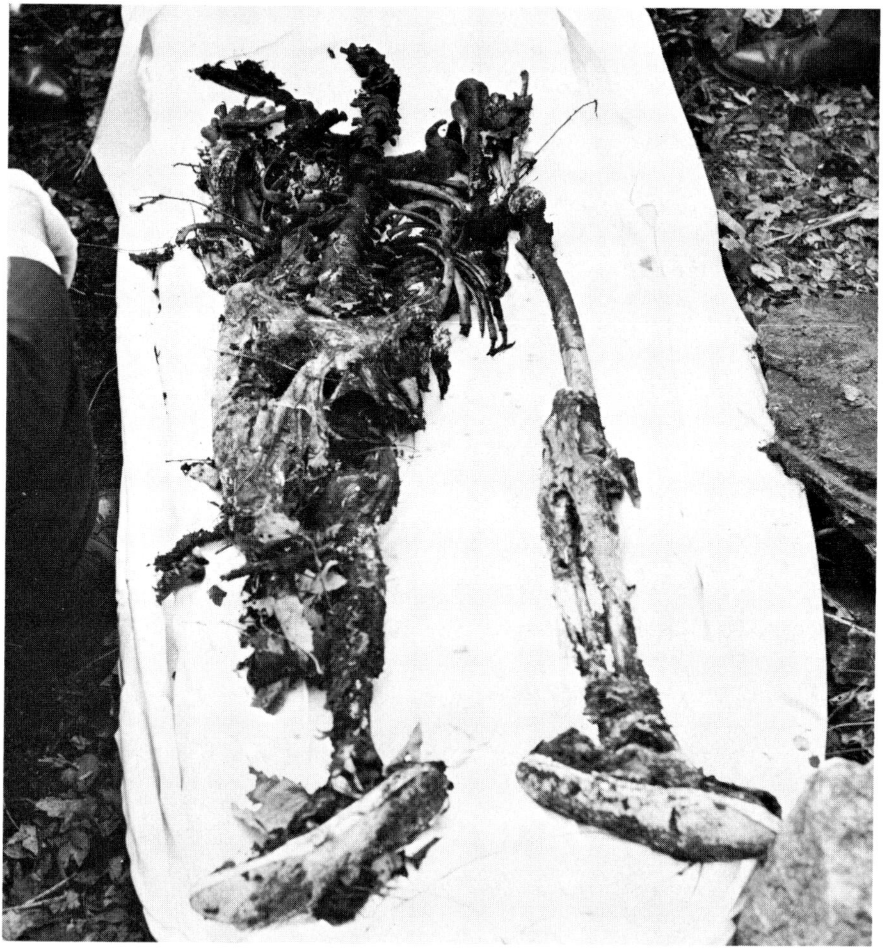

Fig. 15. Headless skeleton, wearing sneakers, found after an anonymous telephone call. (Connecticut State Police)

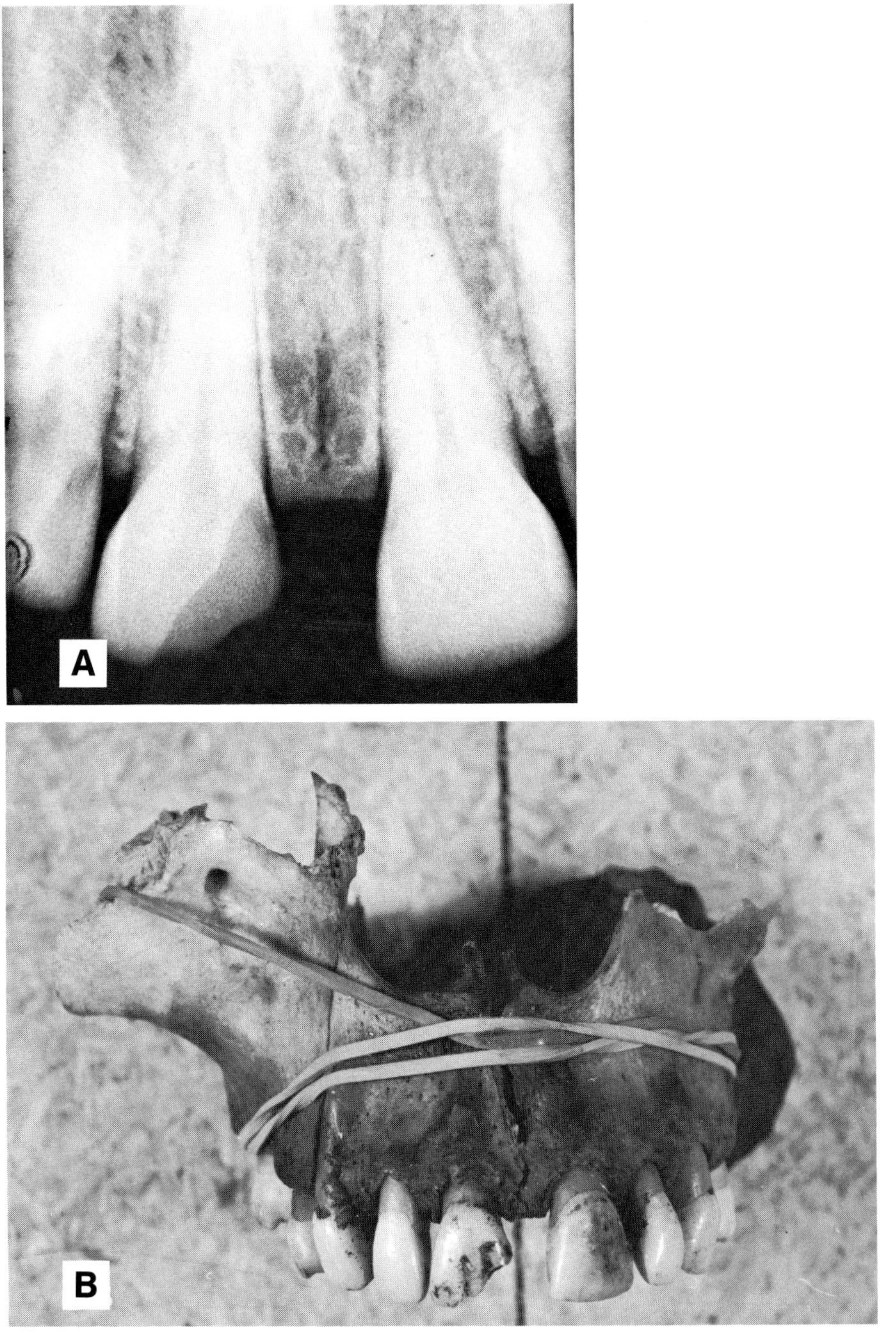

Fig. 16. A, Antemortem x-ray of upper first incisors shows a mesial incisal fracture, *B,* also seen in maxilla of victim.

GLOSSARY OF DENTAL TERMS

ABUTMENT. A tooth used for support or anchorage of a fixed bridge or partial denture.

ACRYLIC. Refers to the plastic methyl methacrylate.

ALGINATE. A material used for taking dental impressions: an irreversible hydrocolloid.

ALVEOLAR BONE. The supporting bone for the teeth.

ALVEOLUS. The bony socket in which a tooth is fixed.

AMALGAM. A dental filling material consisting of silver alloy mixed with mercury.

ANATOMICAL LANDMARK. A prominent feature of the anatomy, such as the nose, eyes, nipples, navel, etc.

ANTEMORTEM. Before death.

ANTERIOR. In the front part of; in front of.

APEX. The tip of the root of a tooth.

ARCH. The curve of the dentition in a jaw.

ARMAMENTARIUM, ARMARIUM. All of the instruments, equipment and other supplies that are used by the forensic dentist.

ARTICULATE. To mount the maxillary and mandibular models in a movable relationship proper to them.

ASPIRATE. To remove by suction.

BICUSPID. A tooth with two projections (cusps) on the chewing surface, also called premolar. There are eight bicuspids in the adult mouth, positioned fourth and fifth to the right and left of the midline in each jaw.

BLOCK. A section of two or more mineral (porcelain) teeth carved and baked as one piece, now an antiquated technique.

BRIDGE, BRIDGEWORK. *See* fixed bridge.

BUCCAL SURFACE. Surface toward the cheek.

CANINE FOSSA. A depression on the external surface of the upper jaw above each cuspid tooth.

CARIES. Tooth decay.

CARIOUS LESION. An area of decay in a tooth.

CAST. *See* model.

CLASP. A thin metal, or plastic, band fitted to a natural tooth to retain a partial denture in place.

COLD STERILIZATION. Chemical sterilization.

COMMISSURE. The corner at each side of the mouth where the upper and lower lips meet.

CROWN. The enamel-covered part of a tooth, normally seen above the gumline, or a replacement for that part, made of gold, porcelain, plastic, stainless steel or a combination of them.

CUSP. A tapering projection on the chewing surface of the back teeth (multicusped) and on the biting surface of the cuspids.

CUSPID. A tooth with one cusp, also called canine. There are four cuspids in the mouth, positioned third to the right and left of the midline in each jaw.

DDS. Dental Disaster Squad, a group of dentists organized to conduct dental identifications following a mass disaster.

DENTAL NOTATION. A system using symbols to designate the teeth and their respective location in the mouth.

DENTAL STONE. A nonporous form of calcined gypsum used for pouring models. It is harder and denser than plaster of Paris.

DENTITION. The kind, number and arrangement of the teeth.

DENTURE. A removable appliance containing one or more artificial teeth replacing natural teeth.

DID. Dental identification.

DISARTICULATE. To separate at a joint.

DISTAL. Away from the midline of the mouth.

EDENTULOUS. Without natural teeth.

ENDODONTIST. A dentist who specializes in the treatment of the nerve chamber and root canal of a tooth.

ERUPTED TOOTH. A tooth that has come through the gum into the mouth.

FACIAL SURFACE. Surface toward the cheek or lips.

FILM PACKET. A bite-wing, periapical or occlusal x-ray enclosed in a light-tight covering that is removed at time of developing.

FISSURE. A crack or fault in the tooth enamel caused by imperfect development.

FIXED BRIDGE. A dental appliance consisting of one or more artificial teeth supported by natural teeth and unremovable by the patient.

FORENSIC DENTIST (ODONTOLOGIST). A dentist qualified in the field of dental identification.

FORENSIC DENTISTRY (ODONTOLOGY). The science of dentistry as it relates to the law.

FULL DENTURE. A removable set of artificial teeth replacing all of the natural teeth in a jaw.

HISTOLOGICAL. Refers to the microscopic study of the structure of tissues.

IMPACTED TOOTH. A tooth below the gumline and prevented from coming into the mouth.
IMPRESSION. A hollow imprint of the mouth or a part of it, made of plaster, wax, alginate or other dental material.
INCISAL. Refers to the biting edge of the front teeth (cuspids and incisors) in each jaw.
INCISOR. Any of the four center front teeth in each jaw.
INFERIOR BORDER. Lower edge, as of the mandible.
IN SITU. In the normal position of a body part.
LABIAL PLATE. The outer bony surface of the jaw.
LABIAL SURFACE. Surface toward the lips.
LINGUAL SURFACE. Surface toward the tongue.
MALOCCLUSION. An irregular alignment of the teeth, jaws or both.
MANDIBLE. The lower jaw.
MASSETER. Either of the cheek muscles that raise the lower jaw in chewing, etc.
MATRIX. *See* mold.
MAXILLA. The upper jaw.
MESIAL. Toward the midline of the mouth.
MIDLINE. The vertical axis in the mouth extending between the two first (central) incisors in each jaw.
MODEL. A reproduction of the mouth or a part of it, made by pouring plastic, plaster, dental stone or other material into a hollow imprint (impression) and letting it set.
MOLAR. Any of the twelve multicusped teeth located in the back of the mouth, three on each end of each jaw.
MOLD. A hollow form in which clay was packed in the construction of a porcelain (mineral) denture, which is now an antiquated prosthesis.
MOLD GUIDE. A specimen set of artificial teeth showing the shapes and sizes of denture teeth produced by a manufacturer.
MOLD NUMBER. The number, letter or combination of them used by a manufacturer to designate a specific size and shape of artificial tooth.
OCCLUSAL. Refers to the chewing surface of the back teeth (bicuspids and molars) in each jaw.
OCCLUSAL PLANE. *See* plane of occlusion.
OCCLUSION. The upper and lower teeth in contact.
ODONTOLOGIST. *See* forensic dentist.
OPERATIVE WORK (DENTISTRY). Deals with the restoration of teeth, usually by means of fillings or crowns.

ORAL SURGEON. A dentist who specializes in dental surgery.
ORIFICE. An opening.
ORTHODONTIST. A dentist who specializes in the prevention and correction of irregular relationships of the teeth and jaws.
PARTIAL DENTURE. A removable dental appliance replacing one or more, but not all, of the natural teeth in a jaw.
PARTIALLY IMPACTED TOOTH. A tooth partly through the gum but prevented from coming fully into the mouth.
PERIODONTIST. A dentist who specializes in the treatment of the tissue around the teeth.
PIT. A pointed depression in the enamel of a tooth due to imperfect development.
PLANE OF OCCLUSION. An imaginary surface (plane) containing the chewing and biting surfaces of the upper and lower teeth when they are in contact. When they are not in contact, another occlusal plane is formed by the chewing and biting surfaces of the teeth in the lower jaw.
PONTIC. An artificial tooth on a fixed bridge.
POSTERIOR. At the back; behind.
PORCELAIN. A tooth-colored material consisting mainly of kaolin, feldspar and flux, as used in modern dentistry for denture teeth, jacket crowns and bridgework—different from the clay composition used in nineteenth century mineral (porcelain) teeth.
POSTMORTEM. After death.
PROSTHESIS. A dental appliance replacing one or more natural teeth.
RADIOGRAPH. An x-ray film.
RAMUS. The perpendicular extension at each end of the lower jawbone.
RESECT. To cut out a section of.
RESTORATION. A dental filling of gold, amalgam or other material or a crown, used to replace lost tooth structure.
RIDGE LAP. The part of an artificial tooth which is embedded in the denture base.
ROENTGENOGRAM. An x-ray film.
RUGAE. Raised folds of soft tissue on the roof of the mouth just behind the front teeth.
RUBBER BASE FORMER. A mold used to shape the foundation when a model is poured.
SDS. Summons Data Sheet, a questionnaire pertaining to the dental investigation of a case.

SHADE GUIDE. A specimen set of artificial teeth showing the color gradations of denture teeth available from a manufacturer.

SHADE NUMBER. The number, letter or combination of them used by a manufacturer to designate a particular color of artificial tooth.

SILICONE. A modern material used for taking accurate dental impressions: a liquid rubber polymer that, when mixed with a reactor, forms a solid rubber.

SWAGE. To shape metal by hammering it against a die.

TEMPOROMANDIBULAR JOINT. The movable juncture of the mandible and temporal bone on either side of the skull.

UNERUPTED TOOTH. A tooth that has not yet come through the gum.

UNIT. A natural or artificial tooth that is part of a fixed bridge.

WAX CARVING, WAX-UP. The gum and teeth shaped in wax as a model for a mineral (porcelain) denture, which is now an antiquated prosthesis.

WEAR FACET. Worn area on a tooth, usually caused by abrasion.

Index